INTERPROFESSIONAL EDUCATION
for COLLABORATION

Learning How to Improve Health from
Interprofessional Models Across the
Continuum of Education to Practice

WORKSHOP SUMMARY

Patricia A. Cuff, *Rapporteur*

Global Forum on Innovation in Health Professional Education

Board on Global Health

INSTITUTE OF MEDICINE
OF THE NATIONAL ACADEMIES

THE NATIONAL ACADEMIES PRESS
Washington, D.C.
www.nap.edu

THE NATIONAL ACADEMIES PRESS 500 Fifth Street, NW Washington, DC 20001

NOTICE: The workshop that is the subject of this report was approved by the Governing Board of the National Research Council, whose members are drawn from the councils of the National Academy of Sciences, the National Academy of Engineering, and the Institute of Medicine.

This activity was supported by contracts between the National Academy of Sciences and the Academic Consortium for Complementary and Alternative Health Care, the Academic Council of the Academy of Nutrition and Dietetics, Academic Council of the American Physical Therapy Association, the Accreditation Council for Graduate Medical Education, the Aetna Foundation, the Alliance for Continuing Education in the Health Professions, the American Academy of Family Physicians, the American Academy of Nursing, the American Association of Colleges of Nursing, the American Association of Colleges of Osteopathic Medicine, the American Association of Colleges of Pharmacy, the American Association of Nurse Anesthetists, the American Association of Nurse Practitioners, the American Board of Family Medicine, the American Board of Internal Medicine, the American Board of Obstetrics and Gynecology, the American Board of Pediatrics, the American College of Nurse-Midwives, the American College of Obstetricians and Gynecologists, the American Dental Education Association, the American Medical Association, the American Occupational Therapy Association, the American Psychological Association, the American Society for Nutrition, the American Speech-Language-Hearing Association, the Association of American Medical Colleges, the Association of American Veterinary Medical Colleges, the Association of Schools of the Allied Health Professions, the Association of Schools and Programs of Public Health, Atlantic Philanthropies, the Bill & Melinda Gates Foundation, China Medical Board, Council of Academic Programs in Communication Sciences and Disorders, the European Forum for Primary Care, Ghent University, the John A. Hartford Foundation, the John E. Fogarty International Center, the Josiah Macy Jr. Foundation, Kaiser Permanente, the National Academies of Practice, the National Association of Social Workers, the National Board for Certified Counselors and Affiliates, Inc., the National League for Nursing, the National Organization of Associate Degree Nursing, the Physician Assistant Education Association, the Robert Wood Johnson Foundation, the Society for Simulation in Healthcare, the Uniformed Services University of the Health Sciences, and the Veterans Health Administration. The views presented in this publication do not necessarily reflect the views of the organizations or agencies that provided support for the activity.

International Standard Book Number-13: 978-0-309-26349-8
International Standard Book Number-10: 0-309-26349-2

Additional copies of this workshop summary are available for sale from the National Academies Press, 500 Fifth Street, NW, Keck 360, Washington, DC 20001; (800) 624-6242 or (202) 334-3313; http://www.nap.edu.

For more information about the Institute of Medicine, visit the IOM home page at: **www. iom.edu.**

The serpent has been a symbol of long life, healing, and knowledge among almost all cultures and religions since the beginning of recorded history. The serpent adopted as a logotype by the Institute of Medicine is a relief carving from ancient Greece, now held by the Staatliche Museen in Berlin.

Suggested citation: IOM (Institute of Medicine). 2013. *Interprofessional education for collaboration: Learning how to improve health from interprofessional models across the continuum of education to practice: Workshop summary.* Washington, DC: The National Academies Press.

"Knowing is not enough; we must apply.
Willing is not enough; we must do."
—Goethe

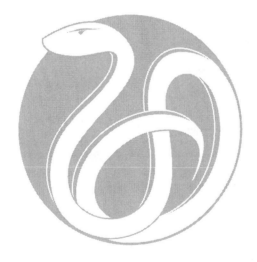

INSTITUTE OF MEDICINE
OF THE NATIONAL ACADEMIES

Advising the Nation. Improving Health.

THE NATIONAL ACADEMIES
Advisers to the Nation on Science, Engineering, and Medicine

The **National Academy of Sciences** is a private, nonprofit, self-perpetuating society of distinguished scholars engaged in scientific and engineering research, dedicated to the furtherance of science and technology and to their use for the general welfare. Upon the authority of the charter granted to it by the Congress in 1863, the Academy has a mandate that requires it to advise the federal government on scientific and technical matters. Dr. Ralph J. Cicerone is president of the National Academy of Sciences.

The **National Academy of Engineering** was established in 1964, under the charter of the National Academy of Sciences, as a parallel organization of outstanding engineers. It is autonomous in its administration and in the selection of its members, sharing with the National Academy of Sciences the responsibility for advising the federal government. The National Academy of Engineering also sponsors engineering programs aimed at meeting national needs, encourages education and research, and recognizes the superior achievements of engineers. Dr. C. D. Mote, Jr., is president of the National Academy of Engineering.

The **Institute of Medicine** was established in 1970 by the National Academy of Sciences to secure the services of eminent members of appropriate professions in the examination of policy matters pertaining to the health of the public. The Institute acts under the responsibility given to the National Academy of Sciences by its congressional charter to be an adviser to the federal government and, upon its own initiative, to identify issues of medical care, research, and education. Dr. Harvey V. Fineberg is president of the Institute of Medicine.

The **National Research Council** was organized by the National Academy of Sciences in 1916 to associate the broad community of science and technology with the Academy's purposes of furthering knowledge and advising the federal government. Functioning in accordance with general policies determined by the Academy, the Council has become the principal operating agency of both the National Academy of Sciences and the National Academy of Engineering in providing services to the government, the public, and the scientific and engineering communities. The Council is administered jointly by both Academies and the Institute of Medicine. Dr. Ralph J. Cicerone and Dr. C. D. Mote, Jr., are chair and vice chair, respectively, of the National Research Council.

www.national-academies.org

PLANNING COMMITTEE FOR EDUCATING FOR PRACTICE WORKSHOP SERIES[1]

LUCINDA MAINE (*Co-Chair*), American Association of Colleges of Pharmacy
SCOTT REEVES (*Co-Chair*), University of California, San Francisco
MALCOLM COX, Veterans Health Administration
JAN DE MAESENEER, Ghent University
MADELINE SCHMITT, American Academy of Nursing
HARRISON SPENCER, Association of Schools and Programs of Public Health
GEORGE THIBAULT, Josiah Macy Jr. Foundation
BRENDA ZIERLER, University of Washington
SANJAY ZODPEY, Public Health Foundation of India

---

[1] Institute of Medicine planning committees are solely responsible for organizing the workshop, identifying topics, and choosing speakers. The responsibility for the published workshop summary rests with the workshop rapporteur and the institution.

GLOBAL FORUM ON INNOVATION IN
HEALTH PROFESSIONAL EDUCATION[1]

JORDAN COHEN (*Co-Chair*), George Washington University
AFAF MELEIS (*Co-Chair*), University of Pennsylvania
KENN APEL, Council of Academic Programs in Communication Sciences and Disorders
CAROL ASCHENBRENER, Association of American Medical Colleges
GILLIAN BARCLAY, Aetna Foundation
MARY BARGER, American College of Nurse-Midwives
TIMI AGAR BARWICK, Physician Assistant Education Association
GERALDINE BEDNASH, American Association of Colleges of Nursing
CYNTHIA BELAR, American Psychological Association
JOANNA CAIN, University of Massachusetts School of Medicine
CAROL CARRACCIO, American Board of Pediatrics (until February 2013)
LINDA CASSER, Association of Schools and Colleges of Optometry
LINCOLN CHEN, China Medical Board
YUANFANG CHEN, Peking Union Medical College
MARILYN CHOW, Kaiser Permanente
ELIZABETH CLARK, National Association of Social Workers
THOMAS CLAWSON, National Board for Certified Counselors and Affiliates, Inc.
DARLA COFFEY, Council on Social Work Education
MALCOLM COX, Veterans Health Administration
JAN DE MAESENEER, Ghent University
MARIETJIE DE VILLIERS, Stellenbosch University
JAMES G. FOX, Association of American Veterinary Medical Colleges
ROGER GLASS, John E. Fogarty International Center
ELIZABETH GOLDBLATT, Academic Consortium for Complementary and Alternative Health Care
MARY JO GOOLSBY, American Academy of Nurse Practitioners (until May 2013)
YUANZHI GUAN, Peking Union Medical College
NEIL HARVISON, American Occupational Therapy Association
DOUGLAS HEIMBURGER, American Society for Nutrition
JOHN HERBOLD, National Academies of Practice
ERIC HOLMBOE, American Board of Internal Medicine
PAMELA JEFFRIES, Johns Hopkins University School of Nursing
RICK KELLERMAN, American Academy of Family Physicians
KATHRYN KOLASA, Academy of Nutrition and Dietetics

---

[1] Institute of Medicine forums and roundtables do not issue, review, or approve individual documents. The responsibility for the published workshop summary rests with the workshop rapporteur and the institution.

vii

JOHN KUES, Alliance for Continuing Education in the Health Professions
MARYJOAN LADDEN, Robert Wood Johnson Foundation
LUCINDA MAINE, American Association of Colleges of Pharmacy
BEVERLY MALONE, National League for Nursing
BETH MANCINI, Society for Simulation in Healthcare
DAMON MARQUIS, Alliance for Continuing Education in the Health
    Professions (until July 2013)
LEMMIETTA G. McNEILLY, American Speech-Language-Hearing Association
DONNA MEYER, National Organization of Associate Degree Nursing
FITZHUGH MULLAN, George Washington University
THOMAS NASCA, Accreditation Council for Graduate Medical Education
ANDRE-JACQUES NEUSY, THENet
WARREN NEWTON, American Board of Family Medicine
KELLY WILTSE NICELY, American Association of Nurse Anesthetists
LIANA ORSOLINI, Robert Wood Johnson Foundation Health Policy Fellows
RAJATA RAJATANAVIN, Mahidol University
SCOTT REEVES, University of California, San Francisco
EDWARD SALSBERG, Health Resources and Services Administration, U.S.
    Department of Health and Human Services (until September 2013)
MADELINE SCHMITT, American Academy of Nursing
NELSON SEWANKAMBO, Makerere University College of Health Sciences
STEPHEN SHANNON, American Association of Colleges of Osteopathic
    Medicine
SUSAN SKOCHELAK, American Medical Association
HARRISON SPENCER, Association of Schools and Programs of Public Health
RICK TALBOTT, Association of Schools of the Allied Health Professions
GEORGE THIBAULT, Josiah Macy Jr. Foundation
JAN TOWERS, American Academy of Nurse Practitioners
RICHARD VALACHOVIC, American Dental Education Association
SARITA VERMA, University of Toronto
PATRICIA HINTON WALKER, Uniformed Services University of the Health
    Sciences
SHANITA WILLIAMS, Health Resources and Services Administration, U.S.
    Department of Health and Human Services
HOLLY WISE, Academic Council of the American Physical Therapy
    Association
BRENDA ZIERLER, University of Washington
SANJAY ZODPEY, Public Health Foundation of India

IOM Staff

PATRICIA A. CUFF, Senior Program Officer

Reviewers

This workshop summary has been reviewed in draft form by individuals chosen for their diverse perspectives and technical expertise, in accordance with procedures approved by the National Research Council's Report Review Committee. The purpose of this independent review is to provide candid and critical comments that will assist the institution in making its published workshop summary as sound as possible and to ensure that the workshop summary meets institutional standards for objectivity, evidence, and responsiveness to the study charge. The review comments and draft manuscript remain confidential to protect the integrity of the process. We wish to thank the following individuals for their review of this workshop summary:

HUGH BARR, University of Westminster, UK
JOHN R. FINNEGAN, JR., University of Minnesota School of Public Health
JILL THISTLETHWAITE, Mayne Medical School, Australia
BRENDA ZIERLER, University of Washington

Although the reviewers listed above have provided many constructive comments and suggestions, they did not see the final draft of the workshop summary before its release. The review of this workshop summary was overseen by **Terry T. Fulmer**, Northeastern University. Appointed by the Institute of Medicine, she was responsible for making certain that an independent examination of this workshop summary was carried out in accordance with institutional procedures and that all review comments were carefully considered. Responsibility for the final content of this workshop summary rests entirely with the author and the institution.

Preface

A century after Flexner, Goldmark, and Welsh-Rose revolutionized postsecondary education for health professionals, two significant reports from the *Lancet* and the Institute of Medicine (IOM) sought to similarly redesign the education of health professionals for the 21st century. The independent Lancet Commission led by Julio Frenk and Lincoln Chen released *Health Professionals for a New Century: Transforming Education to Strengthen Health Systems in an Interdependent World*. The IOM produced *The Future of Nursing: Leading Change, Advancing Health*. Both of these reports provide high-level visions for the health professions, but rely on educators to identify, through a process of continuous learning and innovation, the relevant best practices and mechanisms for scaling up proven, improved approaches to integrated health professional education.

To facilitate the implementation of the recommendations from the IOM and Lancet Commission reports, the IOM created an ongoing, evidence-based forum for multidisciplinary exchanges on innovative health professional education initiatives. Known as the Global Forum on Innovation in Health Professional Education, this forum not only convenes stakeholders to illuminate contemporary issues in health professional education, but it also supports an ongoing, innovative mechanism to incubate and evaluate new ideas—a mechanism that is multifocal, multidisciplinary, and global.

Members of the Forum represent multiple government agencies, industry, academia, foundations, and professional associations. They are drawn from developed and developing countries and come together twice yearly for Forum-sponsored workshops. These workshops provide a platform for relationship building across disciplines and sectors. Such diversity within the Forum is an essential ingredient for innovation and creativity. With 59 members from 16 disciplines and 8 countries, the Global Forum is well positioned to be a catalyst for positive change. Members are committed to breaking down professional silos that impede communication and cooperation among health educators and health professionals and to addressing issues of social justice and health equity around the globe. In our first two workshops, members of our Forum sought to address "interprofessional education." The specific interest was in better understanding the relationships between education and practice in hopes of ultimately improving patient care, advancing population health, and increasing the value of the entire health system.

We would like to thank all those who made the workshops and this Forum possible. Without our sponsors, none of this could have happened. We would also like to thank the planning committee and, in particular, the co-chairs Lucinda Maine and Scott Reeves, who adeptly assisted IOM staff in pulling together two fantastic workshop agendas. We express our deepest appreciation to IOM interns Audrey Avila, Nikita Srinivasan, and Christen Woods for their support; to IOM staff members Patricia Cuff, Megan Perez, and Rachel Taylor for their expert guidance; and to Patrick Kelley for his superb leadership as the director of the Board on Global Health.

This report is a summary of what took place at our 2012 Forum-sponsored events and is a testament to the hard work and dedication of all who make up the Global Forum on Innovation in Health Professional Education.

Jordan Cohen, *Forum Co-Chair*
Afaf Meleis, *Forum Co-Chair*

Contents

1

Introduction[1]

On the morning of July 2, 1881, Charles Julius Guiteau paced nervously around the now-demolished Baltimore and Potomac train depot in Washington, DC, with his newly purchased revolver held snugly in his possession. The unwitting President Garfield, on his way to Williamstown, Massachusetts, for a college reunion, met with two of Guiteau's bullets as he crossed the station preparing to board the train. The first bullet grazed his arm while the second struck him in the back, completely missing his spinal cord. Neither wound was life threatening. But, as was the norm for physicians of the day, a lack of sterile technique resulted in overwhelming sepsis as doctors repeatedly attempted to locate and remove the bullet from Garfield's back using their fingers and unwashed probing devices. Garfield died 11 weeks later weighing 80 pounds less than when he entered the train station that fateful morning (CBS News, 2012; Millard, 2011).

This was the setting within which Abraham Flexner sought to redesign the medical educational system with his 1910 *Flexner Report*. That report formed the foundation for medical education as it was needed in the early 20th century. During that time, Goldmark and Welch-Rose published two other reports that had a similar impact, revolutionizing nursing and public health education, respectively.

Much of the landscape has changed over the past 100 years with regard

---

[1] The planning committee's role was limited to planning and convening the workshop. The views contained in the report are those of individual workshop participants and do not necessarily represent the views of all workshop participants, the planning committee, or the Institute of Medicine.

to the health professions and the setting within which these professionals work. First, there are many more types of health specialists addressing the treatment and prevention of disease. When contributions from each specialty field are well coordinated, the individual person or patient benefits from the communication among all the providers, resulting in improved health and better care as well as less duplication of services and cost savings. Working in this way—keeping the whole person at the center of coordination and education—is advantageous to all and can have particular impact when non-health professionals, such as policy makers, city planners, and religious leaders, assist in delivering specific health messages. These messages can be crafted by representatives of the community with acknowledgment of the important role played by patients, families, caregivers, and nonprofessional and paraprofessional workers, as well as professionals.

A second way in which the landscape surrounding health professionals have changed over the past century is that the demographics of societies have changed through globalization, and the epidemiology of disease has shifted to a greater prevalence of chronic illnesses as many individuals around the world are living longer and adapting to more urban, "Westernized" lifestyles.

Finally, the advent of the Internet combined with greater information access through innovations in technology and mobile devices has made health education more accessible than ever before.

Because of these societal shifts and information-related innovations that have occurred over the past century, changes to the health professions are under way in many parts of the world that are gradually influencing how health professionals are educated. In recognition of the desire for educational changes that better match the needs of the local health care system and of the patients themselves, the global independent Commission on Education on Health Professionals for the 21st Century launched a study on transforming education to strengthen health systems in an interdependent world. This study called for national forums as a way of bringing together "educational leaders from academia, professional associations, and governments to share perspectives on instructional and institutional reform" (Frenk et al., 2010). That recommendation led to the formation of the Institute of Medicine's Global Forum on Innovation in Health Professional Education.

GLOBAL FORUM ON INNOVATION IN
HEALTH PROFESSIONAL EDUCATION

Every year the Global Forum hosts two workshops whose topics are selected by the more than 55 members of the Forum. It was decided in this first year of the Forum's existence that the workshops should lay the

BOX 1-1
Statement of Task

An ad hoc committee of six to eight health professional education experts will plan, organize, and conduct a 2-day, interactive public workshop exploring issues related to innovations in health professions education (HPE). Membership of the committee will involve educators and other innovators of curriculum development and pedagogy and will be drawn from at least four health disciplines. The workshop will follow a high-level framework and serve to establish an orientation for the future work of the Global Forum on Innovation in Health Professional Education. This public workshop will feature invited presentations and small group discussions that will focus on innovations in five areas of HPE:

1. **Curricular innovations**—Concentrates on *what* is being taught to health professions' learners to meet evolving domestic and international needs;
2. **Pedagogic innovations**—Looks at *how* the information can be better taught to students and WHERE education can takes place;
3. **Cultural elements**—Addresses *who* is being taught by whom as a means of enhancing the effectiveness of the design, development, and implementation of interprofessional HPE;
4. **Human resources for health**—Focuses on *how* capacity can be innovatively expanded to better ensure an adequate supply and mix of educated health workers based on local needs; and
5. **Metrics**—Addresses *how* one measures whether learner assessment and evaluation of educational impact and care delivery systems influence individual and population health.

The committee will plan and organize the workshop, select and invite speakers and discussants, and moderate the discussions. A single individually authored summary of the workshop will be prepared by a designated rapporteur.

foundation for the future work of the Forum and that the topic that could best provide this base of understanding was "interprofessional education." The first workshop took place August 29–30, 2012, and the second was held on November 29–30, 2012. Both workshops were structured using the Statement of Task found in Box 1-1, and both focused on linkages between interprofessional education (IPE) and collaborative practice. The difference between them was that Workshop I set the stage for defining and understanding IPE, while Workshop II brought in speakers from around the world to provide living histories of their experience working in and between interprofessional education and interprofessional or collaborative practice.

CONTEXT OF THE REPORT

Because of the close linkages between the August and November workshops, the two workshops are being summarized together in this single report. Both workshops emphasized the importance of engaging students and patients in the dialogue on interprofessional education and also the value of learning from experiences gathered around the world and applied locally. This point was made by a number of the IPE innovators who presented at the workshops and who are cited in the following chapters. These early adopters of IPE formed their programs after studying other national and international IPE initiatives and shared their experiences freely with other participants. This atmosphere of open sharing of ideas and of a mutual genuine interest in the goal of achieving global innovation in IPE set the tone for both workshops and also shaped the approach of this report, which is a modified summary of the presentations and the rich discussions that took place at the workshops. However, it should be noted that, in order to create a smooth flow of the ideas from the two workshops within this one summary report, the report does not follow the chronological order in which statements and presentations were made.

The next chapter begins by describing what IPE is and the value that it adds to societies, universities, education, health, and health care systems as well as to nations struggling with maintaining sufficient faculty for educating students in the health professions. Chapter 3 describes the challenges to initiating IPE. This section is mainly designed to help those individuals seeking to construct or redesign interprofessional education at their schools to learn from the experiences and challenges of others who participated in designing IPE experiences at their own universities. Chapter 4 looks into how educators measure IPE using the currently available tools and how groups are considering new ways of improving these measurements to more accurately assess learners' knowledge, skills, and understanding of IPE. These first four chapters provide the backdrop for the two subsequent chapters. Chapter 5 looks at IPE as part of a larger educational and health system continuum. And Chapter 6 explores students' reactions to IPE and examines what might be learned or gained by engaging patients, caretakers, and communities in improving collaborations and developing interprofessional education experiences. The seventh and final chapter describes speakers' reflections on what they learned and what they heard while participating in the workshops.

REFERENCES

CBS News. 2012. *How doctors killed President Garfield.* http://www.cbsnews.com/8301-3445_162-57464503/how-doctors-killed-president-garfield (accessed March 12, 2013).

Frenk, J., L. Chen, Z. A. Bhutta, J. Cohen, N. Crisp, T. Evans, H. Fineberg, P. Garcia, Y. Ke, P. Kelley, B. Kistnasamy, A. Meleis, D. Naylor, A. Pablos-Mendez, S. Reddy, S. Scrimshaw, J. Sepulveda, D. Serwadda, and H. Zurayk. 2010. Health professionals for a new century: Transforming education to strengthen health systems in an interdependent world. *Lancet* 376(9756):1923–1958.

Millard, C. 2011. *Destiny of the republic: A tale of madness, medicine and the murder of a president.* New York: Anchor Books.

2

Interprofessional Education

Summary: *An overarching theme of this chapter is that interprofessional education provides students with opportunities to learn and practice skills that improve their ability to communicate and collaborate. Through the experience of learning with and from those in other professions, students also develop leadership qualities and respect for each other, which prepares them for work on teams and in settings where collaboration is a key to success. This success is measured by better and safer patient care as well as improved population health outcomes. Although different situations may require different team members, who each bring to the team a unique set of skills, workshop participant Jody Frost emphasized that the patient, the family, other caregivers, and the community are integral members of all teams regardless of the context. These issues and more are described in greater detail below.*

WHAT IS INTERPROFESSIONAL EDUCATION?

According to the World Health Organization (WHO), interprofessional education (IPE) is an experience that "occurs when students from two or more professions learn about, from, and with each other" (WHO, 2010). Although having students learn together can improve the health and the safety of patients, workshop planning committee member George Thibault of the Josiah Macy Jr. Foundation, who provided the introductory remarks to the workshop, emphasized that IPE is not a replacement for education specific to each profession. "This is not about totally smudging together

7

the professions and saying they're all the same," he said, adding that each profession is part of the interprofessional collaboration in order to provide something that somebody else cannot provide. "We still need to rigorously defend and improve the education specific to each profession while we accomplish interprofessional education," he said.

Another important point Thibault raised is that each health profession possesses its own identity and pride in what it does that is special. An interprofessional identity does not replace this, but rather complements the professional identity. Furthermore, Thibault said that IPE is not the only innovation that is needed to improve patient care and health. It is an important innovation which interacts with other educational innovations to improve health professions education, with a goal of improving the health of the public, but it is not a panacea for all health care system problems. There are many other things that require fixing. Sometimes IPE provides a window into what those other problems are (i.e., regulation, reimbursement, workforce), but it alone will not solve those problems.

Thibault also emphasized that experiential learning is a key element of IPE. Experiential learning refers to the practice of students entering a practice environment to better understand how to work collaboratively in "real-life" situations. Thibault also explained that interprofessional learning is different from multidisciplinary learning, in which students from different professions learn or even work in a group. To be truly interprofessional, he said, an interaction requires purposeful integration and collaboration among the disciplines, whether in an educational or practice environment. Workshop speaker Mark Earnest from the University of Colorado echoed Thibault's remarks, saying, "[W]orking in groups is not the same as learning in teams." It was noted by a number of participants that educators and care providers often say they educate or work interprofessionally, but when evaluated, the evidence of collaboration is weak or nonexistent.

As was explained by workshop co-chair Lucinda Maine from the American Association of Colleges of Pharmacy, certain key processes—such as communication, cooperation, coordination, and collaboration across as well as within professions—cut across interprofessional education and can be applied to a variety of collaborative work settings. Participant Jody Frost emphasized the need for focusing on a health professional team that includes all of the health professionals that need to be there along with the patient, the family, the caregiver, and the community. "If we're going to walk the talk," she said, "we need a new language. I would implore us to start talking about change in education and practice around a health professional team rather than a discipline-specific group."

Recognizing the importance of coordinated care in hospital settings, Matthew Wynia and colleagues researched the qualities of well-functioning teams (Mitchell et al., 2012). They found that members of well-functioning teams share an understanding of the team's goals and that each member understands his or her role within the team. Most important, there is a mutual trust among team members. Ensuring clarity concerning roles and goals is a basic principle of well-functioning teams, regardless of the context within which they are working. Wynia, who was a workshop session moderator, stressed that these qualities correspond to tangible inter-professional skills that should be imparted to students. Such skills include practical techniques to make explicit

- the task and goal of the team,
- who is on the team,
- why certain members are selected to be on the team,
- what the role of each team member is, and
- how the members' roles fit together to accomplish the desired goal.

A workshop participant stated that students who internalize these principles through experiential learning with well-functioning teams will be better prepared to participate in similar collaborative care situations after graduation. He said that this, in turn, will lead to clearer team goals and more precise measurements of improvements in health outcomes. The following sections provide examples of meaningful, experiential learning using different modalities through which students can be educated about the qualities of a well-functioning team.

A Social Responsibility for Collaboration

The authors of WHO's 2010 publication *Framework for Action on Interprofessional Education and Collaborative Practice* defined a professional within "interprofessional education" as any individual "with the knowledge and/or skills to contribute to the physical, mental and social well-being of a community." In addressing the social well-being of a community, Sandeep Kishore—who represented one of the student perspectives presented a the workshops—referred to this definition when emphasizing the social responsibility of health professionals to work together to provide optimal services to communities. He went on to say that part of the social responsibility of health professionals is to work together in addressing the "causes of the causes" of ill health that must then be taught to students in an interprofessional manner (see Box 2-1).

Knowing the "causes of the causes" sheds light on the inequalities in living conditions that often shape the quality of people's health and health care. Such "glaring gaps and inequities," according to the commissioners of the *Lancet* report on health professional education (Frenk et al., 2010), "persist both within and between countries." Thibault said that no country

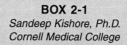

BOX 2-1
Sandeep Kishore, Ph.D.
Cornell Medical College

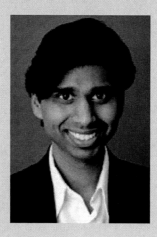

Workshop speaker Sandeep Kishore is a student at Cornell Medical College. His mentors exposed him to data from the U.S. Department of Health and Human Services showing that only 5 of the 30-plus years gained in U.S. life expectancy over the past century were directly due to medical care. The other roughly 25 years gained were the result of improved social conditions, structural development, and behavioral determinants. This realization had a dramatic impact on Kishore's thinking. He began referring to these determinants as the "causes of the causes." It is not just the high cholesterol, Kishore said, but the tobacco addictions, the food addictions, and the policies and structures that influence them. Kishore further commented, "If I'm a health practitioner, a professional who already has an M.D., I'm saying 5 years? That's all we got? This to me has been my pivot to think about systems and change the whole culture of how we work. We can't operate as health professionals alone. We have to reach out to other professions. I would say it's beyond health professions. It's the urban planners, it's the architects, it's the folks that think about inequality. Within health care 5 years is horrific for spending 17 percent of our GDP [gross domestic product] in this country."

is immune from this, including resource-rich nations. In particular, Paul Worley from Flinders University in Australia focused on this point in his presentation, which is summarized in Box 2-2.

Presenters at the workshop offered three examples of interprofessional education grounded in coursework and experiences that teach social responsibility. Jan De Maeseneer from Ghent University described how students at his university learn about social determinants and health inequities by traveling to impoverished communities in Ghent, Belgium, to learn with students from other disciplines. Stefanus Snyman and Marietjie de Villiers from Stellenbosch University in South Africa described how they use the unifying structure of the WHO International Classification of Functioning, Disability and Health Framework[1] (ICF) in clinical care settings to bring different student and faculty professions together around a holistic assessment of the patient. And Elizabeth Speakman described the Health Mentors Program at Thomas Jefferson University, which involves students from different professions learning about the social, cultural, and environmental conditions in which their clinic patients live. Details of each of these presentations are given below.

Jan De Maeseneer, M.D., Ph.D.
Ghent University, Belgium

In the third year of their health professional education at Ghent University, students are exposed to impoverished communities in Ghent, Belgium, to learn with groups of students from medicine, social pedagogy, sociology, and health promotion. Each team explores its assigned neighborhood to observe the characteristics of that neighborhood and the composition of its population. According to De Maeseneer, who is the chair of the Ghent University Educational Committee for the undergraduate medical curriculum, the teams then collect medical data as well as nonmedical indicators such as criminology data, which tell a lot about the quality of life in certain neighborhoods.

Students later come together in a group to discuss the information they collected and observed. This is where culture clashes can arise between medical and social science students, De Maeseneer said, because medical students often want to solve problems immediately, whereas social science students are more apt to analyze the problem, consider the determinants,

---

[1] The WHO International Classification of Functioning, Disability and Health is one of several WHO classifications on health that has been endorsed by the international community to provide meaningful comparisons between and among populations and countries. This tool separates health into four areas: body functions, body structures, activities and participation, and environmental factors. When the four areas are combined, they create an ideal framework for assessing the bio-psycho-social-spiritual health and well-being of a patient.

BOX 2-2
Paul Worley, M.B.B.S., Ph.D.
School of Medicine at Flinders University, Australia

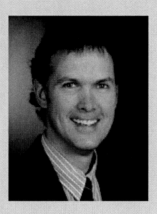

The stark divide between the number of health care workers serving urban Australia versus the number serving rural Australia is striking in every provider category except nursing, whose shortage is seen continent-wide. However, this divide is not just a rural/urban phenomenon; it can also be seen across socioeconomic strata in Australia and around the world, where health outcomes vary greatly by wealth (Marmot, 2012) (see Table 2-1).

Rural Workforce

This is the situation that Worley found when he worked as a doctor in rural Australia. The lack of health providers drove him to the university sector to train and influence future health professionals. His efforts began with just eight students receiving education in rural health clinics. Today, roughly 25 percent of all medical students in Australia are trained in small rural communities rather than in large tertiary hospitals. This is part of a health care transformation meant to graduate roughly 2,000 additional doctors who are prepared to serve rural communities.

Part of the transformational change involved government investment in university departments of rural health with the goal of increasing the rural intellectual capital. Academics would now be based in small rural communities rather than solely in cities talking about small rural communities. Importantly, this investment was described as being not in "rural medicine" but in "rural health," which explicitly demands interprofessional training.

Interprofessional Education

The only way to improve the health of individuals in rural communities is to work interprofessionally. There can be no siloed care. Before the transformation, Flinders University was divided along disciplinary lines. All the doctors were in

TABLE 2-1 Regional Health Disparities for Selected Health Indicators

Region	Mortality rate for children under 5 years/ 1,000 live births (2001)	Infant mortality rate/1,000 live births (2000)	Maternal mortality rate/100,000 live births (2001)	Prevalence of tuberculosis/ 100,000 population (2001)
Developed regions	9	8	20	23
Developing regions	90	63	440	144
Northern Africa	43	39	130	27
Sub-Saharan Africa	172	106	920	197
Latin America and the Caribbean	36	29	190	41
Eastern Asia	36	31	55	184
South-Central Asia	95	70	520	218
South-Eastern Asia	51	39	210	108
Western Asia	62	51	190	40
Oceania	76	66	240	215

SOURCE: Ostlin et al., 2004.

one area, the allied health professionals in another, and the public health clinicians in yet a third. Following the transformation, the structure better reflected the interprofessional research, teaching, and care that the university desired. Six interprofessional clusters were formed. One was the clinical effectiveness cluster, which includes physiotherapists, occupational therapists, orthopedic surgeons, rheumatologists, aged-care physicians, rehabilitation practitioners, and researchers studying the disability sector. These are disciplines that work together in the real world but that are typically trained separately on university campuses. This restructuring challenges the standard hierarchical structure of the university, as the professor of surgery may be supervised in the university sector by a dietitian. It also changes the dynamics and provides an opportunity for understanding how other health providers think.

Benefits of a Community-Based Interprofessional Education

Community Benefits

- University engagement in rural communities: Asking community members to set the program outcomes establishes a direct link between community values and program results. Rural residents appear to value using universities as vehicles to invest in their communities.
- Indigenous participation in medical programs: Rural communities are involved in the selection of the medical students who represent the population being served.

continued

BOX 2-2 Continued

- More rural doctors: Graduates from the rural programs are seven times more likely to choose regional, rural, or remote practices than graduates from a tertiary hospital.
- More primary care physicians: Graduates trained in a primary care setting are twice as likely to choose a primary care practice.

Student Benefits

- A more realistic education: Students learn from the people who make up the population rather than learn about rare diseases of individual patients admitted to a tertiary or quaternary hospital every year.
- Better student scores on examinations: With patients as their teachers, students who learned in small rural communities saw their work as more meaningful. This resulted in these students getting better test scores than students who learned in tertiary institutions despite the exams being set by the tertiary clinicians.

Educator Benefits

- Students serve for the whole year in an interprofessional environment: Students receive orientation for the first three weeks, and then they become productive team members and offer a benefit to those educating them.
- Supervisors have the opportunity to give back to the educational system that trained them and to help form the next generation of health care delivery teams.

Success Factors

The success of the rural interprofessional health education organized by Worley and his colleagues was due to four main factors. The first was the passionate leadership of the clinicians and the second was an acceptance of the work as a "health" alliance rather than a "medical" alliance. A third reason for success resulted from empowering students to be agents of change. Students co-design the curriculum with faculty, which ensures that the curriculum will have greater relevance to them and that they will have greater commitment to the work. The fourth and most important factor was the political campaign from the community

---

and question whether the problem is something that can be addressed by their group. He added that these discussions expose students to different ways of thinking about health predicaments and the thought processes of other disciplines.

Although Ghent University has been offering this community-based experience for 10 years, it has not gotten any easier. Indeed, De Maeseneer

to instigate change. Universities advocating for money for rural health did not have an impact, but rural communities advocating for the government to give money to the universities to do something about the health iniquities was a powerful motivator for change.

Reflections

For a small medical school serving a rural community in Australia, the triple aim may not be the best measure of health from the perspective of the patients in this rural, low-income environment. Much can be hidden within this outcome measure. Improved patient health and even disability-free years are not necessarily correlated with what people report wanting in their lives. People want peace. They want hope. They want love. They want happiness. There is a wealth of research that says health contributes to those feelings, but actually it is quite poorly correlated in many studies (Seligman, 2011). If asked, members of a community such as this may not identify improved health as their ultimate goal. Similarly, improved population health also has faults as an outcome measure of health in rural communities. In Australia overall population health has improved, but the life expectancy of the aboriginal population is 15 to 30 years less than that of the Australian white population. This situation is completely hidden if overall population health statistics are the only outcome measure. Another issue is the strong emphasis on decreasing health care costs when many rural communities may require increased investments, particularly in areas with fewer resources than some high-income areas.

Rural Australia has long suffered from the requirement that it live up to the standard of evidence-based medicine created in—and best suited for—tertiary hospitals. For example, when a patient comes into the emergency department with a headache, the gold standard of care is a CT scan, but this is not the standard in a rural environment, and if a rural clinic fails to meet the higher standard designed for tertiary hospitals, it may be labeled as not providing high-quality care. Similarly, IPE will need to redefine the evidence base used for practice and for quality improvement strategies in various settings. Such strategies are very different in a large hierarchical organization than in a flat, small, primary care system that might have an interprofessional focus.

Finally, no one should underestimate the opportunities for students in IPE to make a difference to health care and to outcomes while they are students, not just in the future. The key is to give learners enough space to be the amazing creative individuals that they are and to develop the relationships with the inspiring people with whom they have to work.

said, the logistics are even more daunting now than they were at the beginning. The experience involves 84 homes that have to be ready to receive the students, 252 caregivers, and 10 community stakeholders as well as tutors, coordinators, assessors, and panel members. "The logistics are really challenging," he said, but clearly not impossible.

Stefanus Snyman, M.B.Ch.B., and Marietjie de Villiers, Ph.D.,
M.B.Ch.B., M.Fam.Med.
Stellenbosch University, South Africa

As at Ghent University, the IPE strategy at Stellenbosch University in Capetown, South Africa, is to educate students through a socially accountable IPE program. Stefanus Snyman, the coordinator of interprofessional learning and teaching at Stellenbosch's Centre for Health Professions Education, said that he sees IPE as a tool for equipping students to become change agents in order to improve patient outcomes and strengthen health systems in Africa. He believes that IPE can be a vehicle for transformative learning and that it is an instrument to foster educational interdependence between the health and the educational systems.

The university's IPE strategy (see Figure 2-1) is based on three pillars and is described fully in Appendix C of this report. The first pillar is the integration of graduate attributes or core competencies into the curriculums and the interprofessional assessment of the competencies. The second

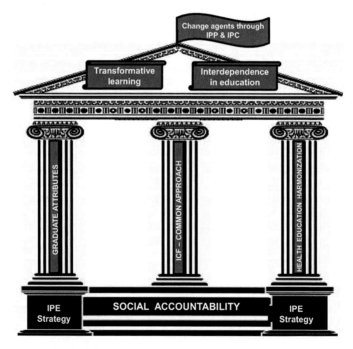

FIGURE 2-1 Stellenbosch University interprofessional education (IPE) strategy.
SOURCE: Snyman, 2012.
NOTE: ICF = International Classification of Functioning, Disability, and Health; IPC = interprofessional care; IPP = interprofessional practice.

pillar is the use of the ICF framework as a common language among all professionals at the school in the management of patient care. According to Snyman and de Villiers, using the ICF Framework in the clinical care setting gives students and faculty a unified structure with which to conduct a holistic assessment of the patient. Under each of the four topic areas (body functions and structures, activities, participation, and environmental factors) are five to nine subdivisions that cover a wide range of health-related issues, including mental function, the cardiovascular system, mobility, self-care, support and relationships, and attitudes. As Snyman said, given the expansive list of assessment items in the framework, no one profession could ever manage the full range of needs identified in a managed care plan. And he added that, in using the framework, students and faculty realize they cannot manage the care of a patient alone and begin the process of working together.

The third pillar is health education and harmonization, which requires leadership from the top as well as learners to make the necessary changes. According to de Villiers, this pillar is designed to equip faculty and community preceptors with interprofessional skills and to develop strategies that bring them together to work collaboratively.

Elizabeth Speakman, Ed.D., R.N.
Thomas Jefferson University

According to Elizabeth Speakman, co-director at the Jefferson Inter-Professional Education Center, the Health Mentors Program at Thomas Jefferson University in Philadelphia has been available to students as long as the university's InterProfessional Education Center has been in existence. This program involves roughly 250 health mentors and roughly 1,300 students from the Jefferson Medical College and the schools of nursing, pharmacy, and health professions, the last of which includes occupational therapy, physical therapy, and couples and family therapy. Each team is made up of students from these different health disciplines, and over the course of 2 years, the students in the teams learn directly from their health mentors—who are patients in the community—about these individuals' health status and living conditions. Speakman said that the work of the students on a team culminates in the fourth and final semester with a visit to their mentor's home in order to experience the conditions and limitations under which their mentor lives.

Following this experience, students are required to write reflective papers. In those papers, Speakman said, students often cite a better understanding of the other health disciplines for their in-depth understanding of the community and the environment in which their patient lives; occupational therapy is often singled out for particular respect because they understand the physical and environmental challenges patients are confronted with outside of the health care facility. Speakman added that students also write about the value of the group leaders who provide guidance on how to communicate effectively with patients and other team members.

Learning IPE Through Patient Safety Activities

Pamela H. Mitchell wrote in the chapter "Defining Patient Safety and Quality Care" that "safety is the foundation upon which all other aspects of quality care are built" (Mitchell, 2008). Linking this notion of patient safety to interprofessional practice, workshop session moderator, Hugh Barr of the U.K. Centre for the Advancement of Interprofessional Education, commented on the recent work of Sexton and colleagues. Those researchers found that improvements in teamwork and culture in intensive care units improved the overall safety climate (Sexton et al., 2011). Using safety as a way to educate students on how to collaborate interprofessionally resonated with a number of presenters at the workshop. Two examples of this approach, from Curtin University and from the University of Missouri, are described below.

At Curtin University, Brewer and Jones developed a framework for IPE curriculum development, which is shown in Figure 2-2. Workshop presenter Dawn Forman from Curtin discussed this framework, which underlies the curriculum and also extends into interprofessional practice. The IPE curriculum starts in the first year, she said, with 23 health professional schools following a model for ensuring client safety and quality. The foundation laid in this first year is built upon in the second, third, and fourth years for each of the programs by having one unit for each profession, which is integrated into each of the subsequent years through workshops, simulation activities, and most importantly, placement activities.

Like Forman, workshop speaker Carla Dyer of the University of Missouri School of Medicine uses IPE patient safety as a way to teach collaboration to her students. She and her colleagues address patient safety and quality improvement using "fall prevention" as the interprofessional teaching modality.

According to Dyer, students first learn about fall prevention through an independent, online study that quickly shifts to a simulation and bedside encounter where students are grouped in dyads consisting of a medical student and a nursing student. The interprofessional simulation first focuses on fall risks in the inpatient setting and then transitions to the home environment. For the bedside encounter, Dyer said, students begin by completing a chart review to gather information about the patient's risk for falls. They

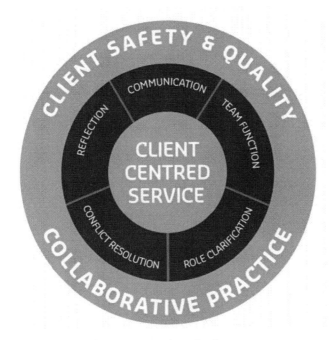

FIGURE 2-2 Framework for IPE curriculum development.
SOURCE: Brewer and Jones, in press.

then review the home environment and the patient care setting. With this information, the students jointly develop a customized fall prevention plan that is discussed with the patient and his or her family member.

Both the medical students' and the nursing students' skills in assessing patient falls are measured before and after their simulation experiences. The results of this assessment showed statistically significant improvements in responses in all of the measured categories, Dyer said. Students were also asked to reflect on the value of the interprofessional experience through an online module; their answers indicated that they valued this experiential leaning opportunity. Program evaluators also wanted to know whether the intervention was valuable to the patients. Dyer and colleagues reported that roughly 250 patients were involved in the simulation activity over the past 3 years and that 93 percent of patients interviewed since the start of the simulation reported that the experience and their interactions with the students were valuable.

Learning IPE Through Community Service

Workshop speaker Gillian Barclay of the Aetna Foundation encouraged the audience to consider interprofessional opportunities that are community-based and that go beyond health. To explain her point, Barclay drew upon the work that Jack Geiger did in the 1960s in rural Mississippi to describe how agriculture specialists engaged with urban planners and health professionals to place farmers' markets near community health centers. She also said the Aetna Foundation is funding evaluation measures within this unique interprofessional space to see how the agriculture experts, the urban planners, the physicians, the managers, and the chief executive officers of these community health centers develop sustainable farmers' markets. This is the sort of culture shift to which students should be exposed, Barclay said, and it was the sort of interprofessional education offered to students in North Carolina under the direction of J. Lloyd Michener and his colleagues at Duke University (see Box 2-3 for a summary of Michener's presentation at the workshop).

Key Messages Raised by Individual Speakers

- Learning in groups is not the same as learning interprofessionally. (Earnest and Thibault)
- An important part of IPE learning is experiential. (De Maeseneer, de Villiers, Snyman, Speakman, and Thibault)
- Interprofessional opportunities that go beyond health can help students understand and address the "causes of the causes." (Barclay and Kishore)
- It is the "causes of causes" of health that need to be addressed and taught to students in an interprofessional manner. (Kishore)

BOX 2-3
Durham and Duke:
A Story of One Community's Journey Toward Health

J. Lloyd Michener, M.D.
Duke University School of Medicine
Department of Community and Family Medicine

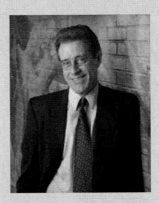

North Carolina is a southern state. It ranks 32nd on the U.S. health rankings and 30th for obesity. One in 10 North Carolinians has diabetes and more than one-quarter of the population is now obese. Trying to deal with these social factors and social issues raises significant challenges, particularly for practitioners at Duke University who provide services to more than 200 sites across the central region of North Carolina. More than half those sites provide primary care.

Community-Based Caring

Michener has been working for more than 20 years in this region of the state. It is a state where the medical home movement has some of its roots and where Michener worked tirelessly with colleagues to improve health care so that the system would be more effective and work better for the communities. Duke now manages networks of Medicaid providers in six counties involving 60,000 people in every primary care site, every health department, and numerous other community groups. To provide the sort of comprehensive care needed in complex societies with complex medical needs, their group required not only committed doctors but also health departments, care managers, dentists, dietitians, health educators, information technicians, physician assistants, nurse practitioners, pharmacists, physical therapists, psychologists, public health workers, and social workers. They also needed the community and its members.

After listening to community needs, neighborhood clinics were built which led to a reduction in the number of emergency room visits, which was a significant savings to the hospital. This led to an expansion of the use of "micro-clinics" in

continued

BOX 2-3 Continued

community "hot spots" with the support of a Federally Qualified Health Center (FQHC) and the hospital because of the significant cost savings.

Practitioners from Duke University are now engaged in a process of slowly weaving health into various aspects of the communities they serve, largely through affiliations with health departments. For example, practitioners work with community groups and health departments to identify safe places to exercise as a way to deal with the obesity epidemic in the neighborhoods. They also staff school clinics, support healthy food programs, and assist with school gardens. In addition, Duke supports access to health information in places of worship and for community groups, and it has provided the funds for community health workers to partner with community members and church groups to spread health information more widely within neighborhoods.

Michener and his colleagues think of their support as weaving health care into the community so that health is actually achieved. The needs of the community dictate who will be assigned to work in an area—with particular attention paid to matching the skill sets of individuals with the needs of an area. The final determination of who provides care is not dictated by who is available; it is determined by what works for that community. In this sense, the Duke program is outcome driven.

Interprofessional Education

Having developed a clear understanding of how to engage with communities and how to provide optimal care that saves money, the Duke University School of Medicine's Department of Community and Family Medicine is now redesigning its educational programs to align student educational experiences with the lessons learned from the department's community engagement. The new curricula emphasize teamwork and collaboration at all levels.

The department offers pipeline programs that expose students in the health professions to community clinics, where they are taught how to work effectively in different cultures. Teamwork is an integral part of this training. There is also a primary care leadership program in the school of medicine that emphasizes teamwork, training, leadership, and improving health outcomes. In this program students do a year of community-engaged research as part of a team.

The Department of Community and Family Medicine is composed of the following seven interdependent groups:

1. Community health
2. Diet and fitness center
3. Family medicine
4. Occupational and environmental medicine
5. Physician assistant
6. Doctor of physical therapy
7. Prevention research

All of the Duke Family Medicine offerings are extremely competitive, and the restructured family medicine residency is no exception, having received 540 excellent applicants for 4 total slots.

Faculty Development

Somewhat unexpectedly, the learners in the department's programs accelerated past the faculty in terms of their understanding of IPE and community-based care. This made it necessary to retrain the faculty. There is now a mandate that all faculty within the family medicine, physician assistant, and physical therapy groups become competent in population health. Currently, faculty are partnering with learners and the community to define the competencies that will then become incorporated into the retraining of faculty members.

Final Thoughts

The work at Duke emphasizes service to the community over professional boundaries. It is the community service that binds the different professions together along with the unified goal of achieving health for all those living in the communities. An important lesson from Michener's experience is that communities vary and that respectful attention needs to be paid to each community's unique history and culture. Communities must be served according to their preference and not that of the professionals working for and with those in the community. This means that what has worked in Durham may not be successful elsewhere. But through active community engagement, other health care systems can be redesigned to improve health and save money along the way. The time to act is now!

REFERENCES

Brewer, M., and S. Jones. In press. An interprofessional practice capability framework focusing on safe, high quality client centred health service. *Journal of Allied Health.*

Frenk, J., L. Chen, Z. A. Bhutta, J. Cohen, N. Crisp, T. Evans, H. Fineberg, P. Garcia, Y. Ke, P. Kelley, B. Kistnasamy, A. Meleis, D. Naylor, A. Pablos-Mendez, S. Reddy, S. Scrimshaw, J. Sepulveda, D. Serwadda, and H. Zurayk. 2010. Health professionals for a new century: Transforming education to strengthen health systems in an interdependent world. *Lancet* 376(9756):1923–1958.

Marmot, M. 2012. Health equity: The challenge. *Australian and New Zealand Journal of Public Health* 36(6):513–514.

Mitchell, P. 2008. Defining patient safety and quality care. In R. G. Hughes, ed., *Patient safety and quality: An evidence-based handbook for nurses.* Rockville, MD: Agency for Healthcare Research and Quality.

Mitchell, P., M. Wynia, R. Golden, B. McNellis, S. Okun, C. E. Webb, V. Rohrbach, and I. von Kohorn. 2012. *Core principles and values of effective team-based care.* Discussion Paper, Institute of Medicine, Washington, DC. http://iom.edu/Global/Perspectives/2012/ TeamBasedCare.aspx (accessed March 12, 2013).

Piroska Östlin, P., G. Sen, and A. George. 2004. Paying attention to gender and poverty in health research: Content and process issues. *Bulletin of the World Health Organization* 82(10):740–745.

Seligman, M. 2011. *Flourish: A Visionary New Understanding of Happiness and Well-Being.* New York: Free Press.

Sexton, J. B., S. M. Berenholtz, C. A. Goeschel, S. R. Watson, C. G. Holzmueller, D. A. Thompson, R. C. Hyzy, J. A. Marsteller, K. Schumacher, and P. J. Pronovost. 2011. Assessing and improving safety climate in a large cohort of intensive care units. *Critical Care Medicine* 39(5):934–939.

Snyman, S. 2012. *Stellenbosch IPE strategy.* Presented at the IOM Workshop: Educating for Practice. Washington, DC, November 30.

WHO (World Health Organization). 2010. *Framework for action on interprofessional education and collaborative practice.* http://www.who.int/hrh/resources/framework_action/en/ index.html (accessed March 4, 2013).

3

Implementing Interprofessional Education for Improving Collaboration

Summary: *Educating formal and informal leaders about the value of interprofessional education (IPE) may be a mechanism for getting leadership support for IPE at the leaders' institutions. This was one message presented by the speaker representing the breakout group on "leadership," and it is a primary focus of this chapter. The chapter begins with the case for why interprofessional education is important, and then it addresses some of the obstacles that implementers may face when promoting or initiating IPE. The discussion includes details on how innovators have overcome or addressed challenges to implementing or sustaining IPE at their universities. In the final section of the chapter, George Thibault reviews some lessons he has learned that could guide future discussions on mainstreaming IPE, which could expand opportunities for students to experience high-quality IPE and collaboration.*

MAKING THE CASE FOR IPE

In the words of Forum and planning committee member George Thibault of the Josiah Macy Jr. Foundation, whose introductory talk addressed why IPE is a key innovation in health professions education, "Interprofessional education is a tool. It's a tool to accomplish linkages between the education system and the health care delivery system. It is a tool to achieve better patient care. It is a tool to achieve better health for the public. It is a tool to achieve a more efficient and affordable health care system." In essence, Thibault said, IPE is a tool for achieving the "triple aim" constructed by the Institute for Healthcare Improvement (IHI)[1] and adapted in this report for use with IPE as follows:

- IPE to achieve better patient care
- IPE to achieve better health (outcomes)
- IPE to achieve more efficient and affordable educational and health care systems

IPE to Achieve Better Patient Care

There is evidence, Thibault said, that care delivered by well function-ing teams is better than care provided by health professionals practicing without coordination (Shortell, 1994; Goni, 1999; Campbell et al., 2001; Stevenson et al., 2001; Mukamel, 2006). There are many examples, he said, of teams that functioned poorly because their members lacked the appropri-ate knowledge, attitudes, and skills. And now more than ever the adverse consequences of poorly functioning teams are causing adverse consequences for many aspects of care outcomes; these consequences include medical errors, inefficient patient care (driving up costs), and a diminished quality of care for patients. Therefore, Thibault said, team-based competencies should be a core goal of health professions education and that some part of all health professions education must be interprofessional. This is the line of reasoning that Thibault stressed in making the case for why education should be taught interprofessionally. As one of the patient representatives at the workshop indicated, patients are the ones who stand to benefit most from improvements in provider communication and collaboration.

Workshop speaker Valentina Brashers, who is part of the University of Virginia's Interprofessional Education Initiative Team, offered an ex-ample of achieving improved patient care through IPE, and she addressed the challenge of bridging the gap between IPE and patient care outcomes. Although it is still a work in progress, she said, the university has taken concrete steps to move IPE from the classroom to the simulation center to the bedside using its Health System Collaborative Care Project (see Table 3-1). This award-winning program offers incentives to health care teams in the hospital setting to develop new models of interprofessional care that involve students at various learning levels. Part of the criteria for receiv-ing these incentives is the inclusion of metrics that ideally include provider outcomes as well as measurements of patient outcomes.

---

[1] The Institute for Healthcare Improvement (IHI) "triple aim" is a framework developed by IHI that describes an approach to optimizing health system performance. It is IHI's belief that new designs must be developed to simultaneously pursue three dimensions—population health, patient experience, and per capita cost—which they call the "triple aim."

TABLE 3-1 University of Virginia Five-Step Model to Advance Team-Based Education and Collaborative Practice

1. Clinically relevant IPE based on collaborative care best-practice models

2. IPE required and integrated throughout the learning continuum

3. Longitudinal assessment of IPE competencies

4. Commitment to continued rigorous IPE research and dissemination of results

5. Bridging the gap between IPE and patient care and outcomes

IPE to Achieve Better Health (Outcomes)

The number of persons with chronic conditions continues to rise rapidly in the United States and around the world, said Forum and planning committee member Harrison Spencer of the Association of Schools and Programs of Public Health, referring to reports from the World Health Organization (WHO) (2011, 2013). If these current world trends in noncommunicable diseases (NCDs) continue, low-income countries are projected to have eight times more deaths due to NCDs than high-income countries by 2030 (Wu and Green, 2000). But "despite the presence of concepts, competencies, rationale, and well-defined need," Spencer said, "public health and its framework of population health have not been integrated into interprofessional education." In Spencer's view, IPE is not about achieving better health, but rather about achieving better health *outcomes*. These outcomes are the end result of a health-related intervention or health care process affecting the health and well-being of patients and populations (AHRQ, 2000). Gaining better health outcomes will require a population perspective, and the only way to achieve positive results, he added, is through more robust funding streams that focus on health outcomes, with IPE as a tool.

Spencer also said that in shifting the focus to health outcomes and population health, one needs to think beyond the acute care setting and to consider less traditional partners from other sectors. He pointed to the model of inter- and transprofessional education (see Figure 3-1) on page 40 of the Lancet Commission report (Frenk et al., 2010) that leads to this sort of broader thinking by including a wider circle of partners, such as community health workers and non-health professions. As Forum member and workshop speaker Gillian Barclay from the Aetna Foundation noted, with such creative modeling comes innovation that resonates throughout the continuum of education and practice.

Spencer said that in population health there are two main sets of partners for IPE that can be drawn from either the clinical professions or from the nonclinical professions. These are not traditional partnerships. As such,

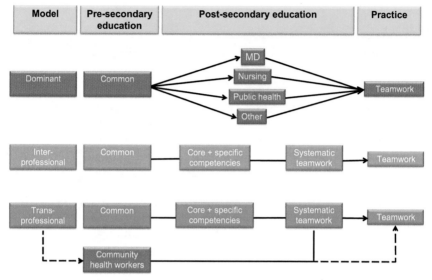

FIGURE 3-1 Models of inter- and transprofessional education.
SOURCE: Frenk et al., 2010.

there is need for new definitions of competencies as well as other relevant details concerning the appropriateness and effectiveness of IPE among the new partners. The issues are summarized in the following two sets of questions posed by Spencer:

Population Health IPE Collaborations with Clinical Professions

- What are the population-level competencies that clinical professions should develop?
- What specific examples of teamwork between clinical and population health professionals can be referred to in developing competencies?
- Are there competencies common to all health professionals in problem solving, communication, and teamwork?
- How do different institutional designs affect the effectiveness of IPE?

Population Health IPE Collaborations with Nonhealth Professions

- Public health is inherently multidisciplinary. Should it be made intentionally interprofessional?

- What are the specific competencies that should be developed vis-à-vis collaboration with lawyers, engineers, economists, policy analysts, urban planners, journalists, and other relevant professions?

In her summary remarks, Forum member and workshop speaker Marilyn Chow from Kaiser Permanente expressed her enthusiasm for the population health perspective, saying that the discussions may have gotten her to rethink whether the core competencies should include competencies related to population health, which would bring to the forefront thinking about the population and the patients as they incorporate public health principles.

IPE to Achieve More Efficient and Affordable Educational and Health Care Systems

Although "start up" funds often are needed to get IPE initiated, once IPE becomes standard practice, educational and health care systems stand to benefit financially through two mechanisms, according to Forum and planning committee member Madeline Schmitt of the University of Rochester. "It seems to me a good part of the costs on the interprofessional side is the cost of going around the silos that we've built," she said. Recognizing the enormous amount of duplication in the content taught in silos is a first step toward cost containment. This recognition does not itself provide interprofessional learning, but it does establish a base from which students and faculty can work together to build interprofessional learning. The second aspect of costs that Schmitt addressed related to the practice side and the need to invest in the retraining of new graduates. "There are real costs associated with that retraining, which we could and should rethink on the education side," she said. This message was aggressively promoted by workshop speaker Paul Grundy, who is the global director of the IBM Healthcare Transformation.

Another way that IPE could decrease costs would be through a decrease in medical errors produced by improved communication. Communication is a cornerstone of interprofessional education, as was emphasized by each of the breakout group leaders' presentations on IPE for "improving health," "providing better care," "enhancing access to education," and "lowering costs." One topic of discussion at the workshop was the high rate of medical errors in the United States, with one participant citing the landmark IOM (1999) report *To Err Is Human*. In that report, published estimates from two major studies indicated that up to 98,000 people "die in hospitals each year as a result of medical errors that could have been prevented"; and, as one speaker pointed out, such medical errors continue today (Levinson, 2010, 2012). Given that the Joint Commission (2012) estimated that 80 percent of all serious medical errors in the United States involve miscommunication, it can be expected that patient safety will improve when students enter the work environment with the superior communication skills that are provided by interprofessional education. As the leader of the IPE and lower costs small group at the workshop, Thomas Feeley of the MD Anderson Cancer Center said that improving outcomes and quality of care lowers the costs of care.

This notion of using IPE to "lower health care costs" did not resonate with all the workshop participants. Forum and planning committee member Jan De Maseaneer of Ghent University in Belgium noted that in many developing countries, spending on health care is minimal and inadequate. Given this situation, he said, the discussion should be about the improved value that IPE could bring to health care in developing countries rather than about lowering costs.

OVERCOMING OBSTACLES TO IMPLEMENTING IPE

George Thibault said that he is a fervent advocate of IPE, although he understands the challenges faced by those implementing IPE programs. The challenges to initiating or sustaining IPE can be logistical, curricular, and cultural and can be more or less difficult depending on the interest of the leadership and the faculty. In his presentation, Thibault laid out a number of potential obstacles to implementing IPE, each of which has been overcome by at least one of the programs in the examples that follow.

Logistical Challenges

According to Thibault, finding the right timing for IPE and the right match of learners among the professions is a concern for planners, as is student engagement in clinical service experiences. Learners want meaningful assignments with real patient care responsibilities, but providing such enriching experiences is difficult when learners are not available consistently throughout the year. To overcome this particular challenge, workshop speaker Dennis Helling, executive director of pharmacy operations and therapeutics at Kaiser Permanente Colorado Region, devised detailed plans for the continuation of the pharmacy service with or without students. In this way, patient care was enhanced by students and was not negatively affected by their absence.

Another logistical challenge that received significant attention at the workshop was the issue of physical space. Workshop speaker Rose Nabirye from the Department of Nursing at Makerere University in Uganda cited this in her workshop presentation. Because she and her colleagues conduct multiple simultaneous small-group discussions of 10 to 12 students, one large lecture hall is not adequate. Her discussion groups now fill any and all available spaces, including professorial offices. Nor was this challenge of physical space unique to Uganda. Workshop speaker Steven Chen from the University of Southern California described space as a "huge issue" for him in his work with students in California at the Safety Net Clinics. As Chen explained, "You do not have a lot of room for all these students. We have had to pair up different disciplines and have different focuses at different visits in order to accommodate that problem."

At the five Department of Veterans Affairs (VA) centers of excellence in primary care education, space has become an institutional issue, according to VA nurse consultant Kathryn Rugen, who spoke at the workshop. She agreed with Nabirye about needing particular spaces for students and not just having them sit in a large room together and listen to a lecture. Specifically, she said, "it has to be an environment where students can have some dialogue and socialize." This was echoed by Forum member Darla Coffey from the Council on Social Work Education, who reminded workshop participants about the importance of having a "social space" outside of the classroom where learning from other professions takes place through thoughtful reflections. "Without this protected space," she said, "the most important element of interprofessional education is lost."

Maria Tassone of the University of Toronto, who spoke at the workshop as the co-leader of the Canadian Collaborative, said that moving from uniprofessional spaces to interprofessional spaces in order to have space to interact is also important for teams working within the practice setting. That idea resonated with workshop speaker David Collier, who directs the Pediatric Healthy Weight Research and Treatment Center at East Carolina University. Collier has found space for clinicians to see patients to be a major issue in his clinic because an initial comprehensive visit could take up to 4 hours. In such situations, working with the manager or others to identify unused office space or to improve the flow of patients, professionals, and students through busy environments like health clinics may help to alleviate space issues—in much the same way as Chen described overcoming the "space" challenge at the Safety Net Clinics.

Curriculum Content

Among the other obstacles to implementing IPE cited by Thibault were knowing the appropriate curricular content and the suitable topics to teach interprofessionally. Another obstacle is knowing how to weave that content into meaningful clinical and community experiences like those set up by Steven Chen at the University of Southern California, which are described in Box 3-1 (page 34).

As was mentioned previously in the summary of Thibault's comments, experiential learning is a critical component of IPE because it is where the imprinting of health professions education takes place. However, imprinting can also take place through a "hidden curriculum" which was identified by a number of workshop speakers. Students may be formally taught to work collaboratively, but within the hidden curriculum, experience educational and health care systems remain mostly siloed. The existence of this hidden curriculum risks sending conflicting messages to students regarding the value of collaboration, said workshop speaker Barbara Brandt from the University of Minnesota. One way to avoid these conflicting signals is to expose students only to well-functioning teams. For example, Brandt described sending students to the Broadway Family Medicine Clinic in North Minneapolis, where they experience a unique culture in terms of both language and behavior. The front desk receptionist leads the staff meeting, and physicians interact fully with nurse practitioners. Although student education is not the primary focus of the clinic, Brandt said, learners internalize the values and behaviors expressed in this nonhierarchical, collaborative environment.

Another technique for dealing with the hidden curriculum was described by workshop speaker Mark Earnest from the University of Colorado. He uses the hub-and-spoke model (described in Appendix D) in which students learn how to work interprofessionally in clinical settings and then return to the university preceptor to discuss their experience. The preceptors tell their students they will learn by negative as well as positive examples of collaboration. A goal of this program, as Earnest described it, is to help keep students focused on the positive examples and to be agents of change to create such environments wherever they go.

Culture

Cultural entrenchment within education and practice remains a significant barrier to collaboration in and across these environments. This was one message from Forum member Warren Newton of the American Board of Family Medicine, who led the small group discussing the initiation of collaborative partnerships. From Thibault, the message was, "We've built up cultures that actually reinforce separation, actually sometimes rejoice in separation and in citing differences rather than the commonality that we have across the health professions with a common goal of improving patient care." Those silos are manifested by poorly aligned calendars, inadequate collaborative space, the perceived lack of time necessary to do interprofessional work, and the need for new models of education, he said. Overcoming these challenges means understanding the different incentives, drivers, and reward systems that exist within the two worlds of education and practice. Once these are recognized, Thibault said, strategies can be developed to break down the traditional professional silos that value independence over collaboration both within education and practice and between them.

External forces sometimes drive cultural changes from traditional, fragmented, discipline-based curriculums to integrated patient- and problem-based curriculums that emphasize interprofessional education. For example, Jan De Maeseener reported how he and medical faculty colleagues were confronted with a very negative assessment by the accreditation board, which pushed them to adapt IPE approaches. Similarly, Nelson Sewankambo reported being forced into IPE because of external circumstances. Despite a 90-year history of providing siloed education to students at Makerere University in Uganda, he and his colleagues introduced IPE in 2001 because of workforce shortages. "We had no choice," he said, because "there was a shortage of teachers and health workers in the country. That is why we went into interprofessional education." In designing the curriculum, Sewankambo worked closely with the Ministry of Health to ensure that graduates entered the workforce with the right set of skills to affect the entire population in addition to the individual communities they served.

IPE innovators around the world may take inspiration from these examples out of Belgium and Uganda and might also consider the idea proposed by Marilyn Chow. She suggested the creation of an entity that is unencumbered by the tradition and bureaucracy of education and health care that could spur a rapid development of new ideas and pilot them through the education and care innovators.

Leadership

Throughout the workshops, an overarching theme was the importance of leadership in bringing about culture change. This point was brought out by Elizabeth Speakman from Thomas Jefferson University (see Box 3-2) and then reiterated by Dawn Forman of Curtin University when Forum co-chair Afaf Meleis from University of Pennsylvania School of Nursing questioned her about the development of interprofessional education at her University. Forman said, "I certainly believe that had it not been for the leadership within the university and also within the Department of Health . . . that interprofessional education would not have been started." Forman went on to cite experiences of universities with IPE programs that were discontinued following a change in leadership. "Leadership is absolutely critical," she concluded.

To determine who can provide leadership and support for IPE, members of the leadership breakout group decided that the first step is to identify the leaders and other stakeholders as well as their relationships to each other and their institutions. The group acknowledged both formal and

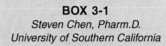

BOX 3-1
Steven Chen, Pharm.D.
University of Southern California

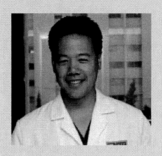

Workshop speaker Steven Chen commented in his talk that three settings where he and his colleagues have IPE students are areas that desperately need help and are prime areas for interprofessional education. These include the safety net system, geriatrics, and psychiatry. In the safety net area, he said, resources like space and supplies are extremely limited and there are very few specialists willing to see the underserved. The primary care providers are heavily burdened to provide great care for those patients, adding that he and his colleagues have seen dramatic shifts in the demographics of patients they serve as the economy continues to struggle. Although Chen said they started with minority patients in most clinics, they now see a wider variety of ethnicities in the clinics with whom they partner.

Literacy, culture, and poverty are major barriers to adherence with medications as well as following lifestyle and self-management recommendations. These barriers frustrate even the most competent physicians, who find it impossible to address all of them adequately for the highest-risk patients. As a result, Chen said it is difficult to retain providers because of the high stress level of the safety net environment. Team-based care, where every member of the team provides services at their maximum scope of practice, provides great value in this setting by addressing patient needs and reducing physician workload and stress.

The first of three student programs Chen and/or his colleagues initiated that involve safety net settings is called SHARE or Students Helping and Receiving Education. It is an 8-year program that offers critical services, such as medication reconciliation and smoking cessation classes, through pharmacy student volunteers, but now engages other disciplines. Chen says this work was aided significantly by the Center for Medicare and Medicaid Innovation (CMMI) grant that is allowing them to integrate clinical pharmacy services into a network of safety net clinics during the next 3 years. Services provided through the SHARE program to other safety net clinics are now being developed for the safety net clinic organization supported by the CMMI grant.

The second program Chen described was the University of Southern California (USC) student-run clinic (see Figure 3-2). The difference between SHARE and the USC student-run clinic, he said, is that SHARE was a student IPE program that was integrated into an existing practice whereas the student-run clinic was created specifically for IPE by students. "This is one of those examples," said Chen, "of 'get out of the way and let the students run it' because they do such a great job."

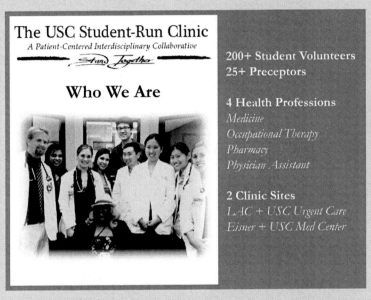

FIGURE 3-2 The USC student-run clinic.
SOURCE: Courtesy of Steven Chen.

Another program that Chen discussed exposes students to team-based care for chronic condition, like asthma. In this example, Chen helps students develop or update asthma education materials that are used to teach a monthly student-run patient education program on asthma management at a safety net clinic. The class is mandated for all patients with newly diagnosed asthma at the clinic and is an integral part of a clinic-wide asthma management program. Students teach about the basic pathophysiology of asthma in simple terms, how to recognize and manage symptoms, what the medications do and how they should be taken, how to use asthma-related devices, and how to measure peak flow. Most patients with very poorly controlled asthma are also enrolled into the pharmacist-run asthma management program. In testing their effectiveness, Chen reported a greater than two-fold likelihood of patients reaching their asthma control goals, as defined by current guidelines, when they are enrolled in the clinical pharmacy program and participate in the asthma education class versus not being involved. Chen attributed the positive results to a combination of hard work by the clinic providers, including the clinical pharmacist, as well as students' involvement.

BOX 3-2
Elizabeth Speakman, Ed.D., R.N., CDE, ANEF
Jefferson InterProfessional Education Center, Thomas Jefferson University

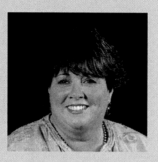

Although many interprofessional activities were occurring at Thomas Jefferson University prior to the establishment of the Jefferson InterProfessional Education Center (JCIPE), presenter Elizabeth Speakman said, the activities were mainly occurring sporadically among different programs. Speakman acknowledged realizing that many faculty champions would be necessary to make it possible to implement interprofessional education the way the early innovators envisioned. Additionally, a way was needed for this vision to be solidified and coordinated through a particular organization. This was the vision of the university president, she said. In 2007, the JCIPE was developed, based on the president's vision, to establish such a coordinating center, which was supported by the deans. It was this unified effort that led to the establishment of a standalone center at Jefferson with its own budget. This independent budget, Speakman said, helps the faculty produce some of the IPE activities offered at the university.

Speakman also said that JCIPE is supported by a very robust steering committee which came together to draft the center's mission and vision. The center has an interprofessional curriculum committee that is headed by the JCIPE but that also includes service providers as well as representatives from library services. All stakeholders from Thomas Jefferson University were invited to come together to review the curriculum being proposed by the committee.

From these reviews it became evident that a framework was needed for the curriculum. In response, the curriculum committee worked on adapting the International Education Collaboration curriculum and came up with four competencies that every Jefferson student would have upon graduation. The next step, which Speakman said she and her colleagues are working on now, is moving toward requiring students to meet these competencies in order to graduate from Jefferson. None of this would have been possible, Speakman said, without the support of the university leadership.

informal levels of leadership and the importance of engaging all leaders as change agents.

Leaders with little IPE experience will require education on what IPE is and the value that it can provide for students, faculty, and, more broadly, the entire health care system. Providing clear and consistent messages, definitions, and evidence is the most effective way to arm the leader with what is needed to advocate for IPE. However, a leader needs to understand that there are different types of evidence. There is initiating evidence used to define the problem, and there is sustaining evidence which is generated continuously to show the ongoing impact being made through IPE.

Those providing the evidence must be cognizant of the different meanings that their data could hold for different stakeholders and be clear about the purpose of the information provided. As Melissa Simon from Northwestern University, the presenter for the leadership breakout group, explained, "There is a flash point. There is a critical mass of the amount of evidence that we build, how visible we become, and what is the economy of scale." Her remarks were sensitive to the challenges leaders face in having to sort through facts for relevant information. When providing evidence, Simon said, it is best to include specifically how, when, and why—and the context within which—the evidence was obtained. The purpose is not merely to convince, but also to build relationships and connections with leaders that involve patients who can demand change and students who are the leaders of tomorrow.

Simon shared other views expressed by many members of the leadership breakout group, which included several expectations for leaders. Leaders must be permissive, encouraging, directive, and explicit while also delivering resources. Additionally, they must model and enforce accountability among others by promoting and sustaining a culture of teamwork and respect. Members of the group also spoke of leaders' responsibility for building champions of IPE through scholarships, publications, and dissemination of current IPE activity outcomes and urged that leaders support capacity-building activities, such as leadership training and interprofessional collaboration. This type of leadership capacity building is exemplified in the Canadian Collaborative described in Appendix C of this report. Finally, members of the group spoke of the need for positive assessment and evaluation outcomes in order to more effectively and fluently convince leadership of the importance of IPE.

Faculty Development

In the closing remarks of his presentation, George Thibault focused on the importance of committing time and energy to faculty development in an effort to decrease reluctance about interprofessional education. This resonated with Nelson Sewankambo, who described how he experienced faculty reluctance to IPE firsthand in 2001 at Makerere University. Initially, he said, faculty were apprehensive about educating students interprofessionally because they themselves were not trained in IPE and understandably felt great discomfort in teaching this way. However, Sewankambo said, many of the faculty members at Makerere who embraced a more holistic approach to health professions education pushed to receive master's degree–level training so they could better understand health professions education. In turn, he said, those faculty members became the advocates of IPE at the university. J. Lloyd Michener, workshop speaker from Duke University, described experiencing a similar faculty excitement over IPE; once the faculty accepted and understood the elements of interprofessional education, he said, they realized the work was "really fun."

At the University of Southern California, Steven Chen reported that one of the biggest challenges to developing IPE is getting faculty to understand what other professions do. This has been addressed by hosting a series of seminars and workshops that run throughout the year. All faculty members who participate in their IPE programs are invited to these events as a way of learning about the other professions in their IPE program. Chen added that when he hosts these seminars, he models them after the Health Resources and Services Administration Patient Safety and Clinical Pharmacy Services and the Institute for Healthcare Improvement's "all teach, all learn" approach.

Gillian Barclay reported that at the Aetna Foundation, the WHO definition of IPE—noted in Chapter 2 in this report—is modified to read "*faculty* from two or more professions learn about and with each other to enable effective collaboration and improve health outcomes." In her opinion, if the students can do it, it is important for faculty to also work and learn in the same way.

Because of the critical importance of a trained staff to providing interprofessional education, most if not all of the IPE programs described at the workshop were reported as offering some component related to faculty development. Across Canada, faculty development is an important feature of IPE, and it is designed for clinical as well as educational faculty. The University of Toronto alone has trained more than 700 faculty members in IPE. Although this seems an impressive accomplishment, Maria Tassone put that effort into perspective by noting that the University of Toronto has 5,000 clinicians, and thus a lot of work remains. Appendix D lists some faculty development programs at various universities.

LESSONS LEARNED

George Thibault commented that the Forum members, speakers, and participants attending the workshop represented an incredible wealth of experience. Everybody had his or her own stories to tell and his or her own biases, he said, and a number of important lessons emerged, dating as far back as the earliest experiences with IPE. These lessons can guide future discussions on mainstreaming IPE and can expand opportunities for high-quality interprofessional education and collaboration. Thibault offered six lessons from his own experience, elaborating on each in turn. The lessons were

1. Leadership from the top is essential.
2. Extensive planning is necessary for rigorous experiences.
3. Experiences need to be repeated throughout the educational continuum.
4. IPE must accomplish real work; it is not an end in itself.
5. New technologies can assist in accomplishing goals.
6. A major commitment to faculty development is required.

Leadership from the Top Is Essential

Although the importance of leadership from the top may be a truism that applies to multiple situations, Thibault said, it has been absolutely imperative for success within IPE. Without leadership from the top, the logistical barriers become obstacles that cannot be overcome. Thibault made the point by noting that deans can change schedules, they can change the reward structure for faculty, they can assign time differently, and they can make resources available. He also stressed that the institutions that have gone farthest with IPE have gotten support at the highest level of leadership, including deans, provosts, chancellors, and presidents.

Extensive Planning Is Necessary for Rigorous Experiences

According to Thibault, some of the early encounters in interprofessional education may have been looked at negatively because they were seen as extracurricular and not truly educational. Socialization is an important part of education, he added, but it is not education in and of itself. The classic high school mixer is not an educational experience, for example. Interprofessional educational experiences need to be planned rigorously with clear educational goals in mind, clear metrics, and measured outcomes, he said. They are not casual encounters.

Experiences Need to Be Repeated Throughout
the Educational Continuum

Thibault commented that even the most thoroughly well-planned single encounter will not have a lasting impact. Experiences need to be repeated in order to overcome cultural barriers, and they need to be reinforced, given the huge volume of information that all health professions students must learn and experience to become fully developed professionals. If IPE is offered only as an annual event, then the message is clearly given that it is not core. To be core, he said, it must be seen as something that is repeated regularly throughout education.

IPE Must Accomplish Real Work; It Is Not an End in Itself

When the interprofessional educational activity is aligned with real-life situations and challenges, Thibault said, the IPE experience becomes more tangible and applicable to real work. Such an experience has a more lasting and enduring impact and is more valued by learners. Designers of IPE need to look for those opportunities that can only be done or are best accomplished interprofessionally, he said. If the activity does not require collaboration and it does not provide real-life experiences, Thibault said, it should not be called "interprofessional education."

New Technologies Can Assist in Accomplishing Goals

Thibault said that technology for IPE is just beginning to unlock the possibilities of how learners are learning and will learn differently. It opens up huge possibilities for interprofessional work, he said, as educators become freed from the confines of the fixed classroom and can think in terms of virtual space for education.

A Major Commitment to Faculty Development Is Required

Finally, Thibault commented that most faculties have not experienced IPE or worked across faculty boundaries. As a result, many educators are uncomfortable with teaching interprofessionally because they do not know what to expect with learners of other professions. The enabling technologies for teaching interprofessionally may be unfamiliar to some educators, he stressed, thus causing the educators greater apprehension about engaging in IPE activities. To overcome these challenges, a major investment in faculty development is necessary, Thibault said. For those institutions that have made the investment, IPE has been an incredible source of renewal in terms of energizing the faculty by teaching them new tools, having them be with students from different professions, and engaging kindred spirits from other faculties. It has proven to be a way of reinforcing the importance of the educational mission and why educators chose to become faculty members in the first place.

Key Messages Raised by Individual Speakers

- IPE is a tool for achieving the triple aim. (Thibault)
  IPE is about achieving better health *outcomes*. (Spencer)
- Recognizing the enormous amount of duplication in the content taught in silos is a first step toward cost containment. (Schmitt)
- There are real costs associated with retraining, which could be rethought by educators. (Grundy and Schmitt)
- The hidden curriculum risks sending conflicting messages to students regarding the value of collaboration. (Brandt)

REFERENCES

AHRQ (Agency for Healthcare Research and Quality). 2000. Outcomes Research: Fact Sheet. March 2000. Agency for Healthcare Research and Quality, Rockville, MD. http://www.ahrq.gov/research/findings/factsheets/outcomes/outfact/index.html (accessed June 26, 2013).

Campbell, S. M., M. Hann, J. Hacker, C. Burns, D. Oliver, A. Thapar, N. Mead, D. G. Safran, and M. O. Roland. 2001. Identifying predictors of high quality care in English general practice: Observational study. *British Medical Journal* 323(7316):784–787.

Frenk, J., L. Chen, Z. A. Bhutta, J. Cohen, N. Crisp, T. Evans, H. Fineberg, P. Garcia, Y. Ke, P. Kelley, B. Kistnasamy, A. Meleis, D. Naylor, A. Pablos-Mendez, S. Reddy, S. Scrimshaw, J. Sepulveda, D. Serwadda, and H. Zurayk. 2010. Health professionals for a new century: Transforming education to strengthen health systems in an interdependent world. *Lancet* 376(9756):1923–1958.

Goni, S. 1999. An analysis of the effectiveness of Spanish primary health care teams. *Health Policy* 48:107–117.

IOM (Institute of Medicine). 1999. To err is human: Building a safer health system. Washington, DC: National Academy Press.

Joint Commission. 2012. Joint Commission online. June 27. http://www.jointcommission.org/assets/1/23/jconline_June_27_12.pdf (accessed on April 9, 2013).

Levinson, D. R. 2010. *Adverse events in hospitals: National incidence among Medicare beneficiaries.* Washington, DC: Department of Health and Human Services, Office of the Inspector General.

Levinson, D. R. 2012. *Hospital incident reporting systems do not capture most patient harm.* Washington, DC: Department of Health and Human Services, Officer of the Inspector General.

Mukamel, D. B., H. Temkin-Greener, R. Delavan, D. R. Peterson, D. Gross, S. Kunitz, and T. F. Williams. 2006. Team performance and risk-adjusted health outcomes in the program of all-inclusive care for the elderly (PACE). *Gerontologist* 46(2):227–237.

Shortell, S. M., J. E. Zimmerman, D. M. Rousseau, R. R. Gillies, D. P. Wagner, E. A. Draper, W. A. Knaus, and J. Duffy. 1994. The performance of intensive care units: Does good management make a difference? *Medical Care* 32(5):508–525.

Stevenson, K., R. Baker, A. Farooqi, R. Sorrie, and K. Khunti. 2001. Features of primary health care teams associated with successful quality improvement of diabetes care: A qualitative study. *Family Practice* 18(1):21–26.

WHO (World Health Organization). 2011. Global status report on noncommunicable diseases 2010. http://www.who.int/nmh/publications/ncd_report2010/en (accessed March 22, 2013).

WHO. 2013. Deaths from noncommunicable diseases. http://www.who.int/gho/ncd/mortality_morbidity/ncd_total/en/index.html (accessed March 4, 2013).

Wu, S., and A. Green. 2000. Projection of chronic illness prevalence and cost inflation. Santa Monica, CA: RAND Corporation.

4

Metrics

Summary: *The importance of measuring impacts from interprofessional education resonated with Forum member and workshop planning committee co-chair Scott Reeves of the University of California, San Francisco. Reeves, who has devoted much of his career to studying the impact of interprofessional education (IPE), said, "If we want to understand culture and begin to develop robust metrics, we need to go in there and we need to study it," he asserted. In essence, implementers of IPE need to be clear about the purpose of their work so that researchers can confidently analyze whether or not a program is successful. According to Reeves, having robust measurements of the effectiveness of IPE allows programs to be compared and conclusions to be drawn. This assertion was echoed by other participants at the workshop and forms the foundation for this chapter on developing metrics to advance interprofessional education and collaborative care.*

EMBRACING A COMMON PARLANCE

Without clear conceptualizations of what is being investigated and without a common understanding of what various terms mean, researchers studying IPE face a variety of problems, Reeves said. He also noted that throughout the workshop participants had inaccurately used some words interchangeably. For example, he said, despite how some participants had used the words, "assessment" is not the same as "evaluation." And although "interprofessional" had been defined early in the workshop, participants continued to mix their terms and offer examples of interdisciplinary and multidisciplinary education and care. Reeves emphasized that one must be clear about the terminology and concepts or the entire research methodology becomes flawed.

Assessment Versus Evaluation

Reeves made a useful distinction between assessment and evaluation. *Assessment* is done to determine the level of understanding by a learner, while *evaluation* is a tool to determine how well a program or an educator teaching a course is conveying messages. For assessment, he says, there needs to be a meaningful analysis of how the individual learns, not just in the short term but in the long term as well. For evaluation, thoughtful consideration is needed to determine how well the program is conveying the desired messages and information.

Interprofessional, Interdisciplinary, or Multidisciplinary

The terms "interprofessional" and "interdisciplinary" are often used interchangeably in the literature, but at the workshop most speakers and participants used the word "interprofessional." This is not surprising, said Reeves, given that the workshop title included the term "interprofessional education." These terms imply an integrative, collaborative approach to education or practice, he said. On the other hand, *multidisciplinary* simply means several fields, areas of expertise, or disciplines coming together without integrating the services (Reeves et al., 2010).

MEASUREMENT PRACTICES IN IPE

According to Forum member Eric Holmboe of the American Board of Internal Medicine (ABIM), there are two overarching themes that arise when one discusses measurement practices in IPE: the need for competency-based models and the need for a more robust evidence base. Although work is under way to fill the gaps in the evidence base, serious obstacles remain because of uncertainty about what to measure and how to measure it.

Currently, Holmboe said, there are differences of opinion regarding what the unit of analysis should be when measuring various aspects of IPE (i.e., individual, programmatic, institution) and where such an assessment should start. One Forum member suggested that, regardless of whether the analysis is of the faculty, the curriculum, the patient, or the community, the tools do exist, but the analysis needs to be broken out in a way that allows tools to be applied.

Analyzing Program Design

A number of workshop participants proposed starting with the desired results and working backward to determine the best ways to educate students. However, Holmboe said, this design goes against most health professional education models, which typically start with the student and work forward. Holmboe added that working this way also means educators have to predict what future practice will entail and to attempt to prepare health professional students to fit within that model. The World Health Organizatin (WHO) International Classification of Functioning, Disability and Health framework, presented by workshop speaker Stefanus Snyman in Chapter 2, may be a useful tool for envisioning such a practice, he said.

Purposeful IPE Research and Program Design

As the leader of the small group on IPE assessment, Holmboe reported to the wider audience the group's contention that before initiating any assessment, the purpose of the assessment should be clarified. If the purpose is to drive improvements and feedback, for instance, tools could be built that have catalytic effects that impel future learning to improve health and to drive education. One example of this is the Kaiser Permanente care teams in Colorado. A care team includes physicians, clinical pharmacists, nurses, and medical assistants. A main focus of the teams' care since 2008 has been hypertension control. During that time the percentage of members who kept their hypertension under control went from 61 to 83 percent, the latter of which is roughly 10 to 30 percent above the national average. As workshop speaker Dennis Helling, executive director of pharmacy operations and therapeutics at Kaiser Permanente, said, "We are a team-based, fully integrated delivery system, with an electronic medical record that is a great site for IPE." And, he added, the pharmacy operations section is taking full advantage of this IPE opportunity by engaging its students in meaningful work as part of these well-functioning teams.

Despite the accepted benefits of student exposure to well-functioning teams like those at Kaiser Permanente Colorado, it has not been possible to directly measure the effects of interprofessional education on health. As Holmboe said, to assess IPE well, researchers will likely need to embrace more complex measurement strategies that require developmental expertise as well as a knowledge of methodology and program evaluation. It is possible, he said, that a combination of approaches and tools that includes both qualitative and quantitative methods will be required.

Holmboe speculated that the argument against a complex approach to analysis would be that it is easier to use the reductionist model of measuring small pieces of IPE. The problem, as he sees it, is that such a simplification inevitably leads to a loss of information, bringing into question the meaning and the value of the assessment. Speaker Mark Earnest of the University of Colorado agreed and then elaborated on the issue. To assess collaboration effectively, he said, one needs measurements that are valid and reliable. He added, to be valid and reliable, the data need to be multi-source (that is, not just from a single person), to occur over multiple points in time across multiple settings, and to be measured against a standardized rubric. This is quite difficult to accomplish, Earnest said, although ABIM is working on developing such a model. Holmboe, who is from ABIM, pointed to the realist evaluation strategy by Ray Pawson and Nick Tilley and also to Michael Quinn Patton's developmental evaluation as approaches that might provide insights into how IPE could be assessed and evaluated (Pawson and Tilley, 1997; Patton, 2011). In thinking through the various models to assess his students' ability to work collaboratively, Earnest said that he studied the pros and cons of various educational models. More details are provided in Box 4-1.

Self-Directed Assessment

Assessment is something that all health professionals need to do to remain relevant within a field, but, Holmboe said, most often the assessor is not the person who would benefit most from the assessment. Thus he suggested that organizations should increasingly move to self-directed assessments. However, he said, this would have ramifications for the measurements of professional collaborative relationships. "When you ask an audience if they collaborate well, everybody puts their hands up, because nobody wants to say they're a bad collaborator." Thus one issue is whether self-assessment is biased and, if it is, how that would impact interprofessional assessment.

One participant from the breakout group on assessment suggested using newer technologies to track self-assessments in a more structured manner. This might include portfolios, blogs, or electronic applications installed on mobile devices, such as iPhones and iPads, which could be sources of information for measuring the effectiveness of IPE applications. In fact, the participant said, some IPE programs are already using blogs within portfolios that capture what happens over time, particularly from a developmental perspective.

Forum and planning committee member Jan De Maeseener of Ghent University in Belgium commented that the IPE instructors at Ghent University require students to maintain a portfolio of written and electronic reflections that begin with their first year and continue throughout their 6 years at the university. The reason for having students' include their clinical experiences in the portfolio, he said, is to encourage them to internalize the need for lifelong continuous professional development.

ASSESSMENT TOOLS

Eric Holmboe, in his presentation about the breakout group he led, talked about the need for faculty who are competent in IPE. "A general problem for all of concept-based education," he said, "is that we have a faculty workforce across all the health professions who were not trained in the very system we are trying to create." Based on the discussions of his small group, Holmboe commented that many faculties are struggling, so it will be necessary to offer many co-learning activities around assessment as well as education.

Despite the challenges to measuring competencies among learners, a number of presenters at the workshop did report the existence of fairly robust tools for assessing learners and evaluating programs at their institutions. The tools reported by the presenters are described below, organized by the universities at which the various IPE measurement methods are used.

Curtin University

At Curtin University in Australia, faculty have developed the Interprofessional Capability Assessment Tool (ICAT), illustrated in Figure 4-1. Drawn from models developed at Sheffield Hallam University and the University of Toronto, the ICAT assesses students within four domains: communication, professionalism, collaborative practice, and client-centered service and care. Students, faculty, and field preceptors all complete the ICAT form to provide students with feedback on the development of their interprofessional capabilities.

University of Colorado

Earnest, the IPE director from the University of Colorado, reported using an assessment program from Purdue University called the Comprehensive Assessment for Team-Member Effectiveness (CATME). With this tool, self- and peer-assessment information is gathered to determine how successfully each member contributed to the team's performance. There are no assessments from individuals provided in the CATME report, only group feedback created by aggregating the data from individual responses. The eventual goal is to be able to compare these outcomes with team performance scores gathered from other interprofessional activities in order to measure their students' interprofessional growth over time.

BOX 4-1
Mark Earnest, M.D., Ph.D.
University of Colorado

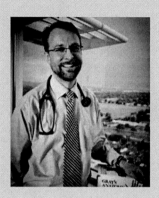

When designing the interprofessional experience for students at the University of Colorado, Mark Earnest and colleagues studied the pros and cons of various educational models. They were particularly interested in finding a model that could assess student learning. Through their research they considered the following models:

- Traditional model of the facilitated discussion
- Group projects
- Problem-based learning
- Michaelson's team-based learning model

In the traditional model of the facilitated discussion, students participate in a planned "experience" and read literature to more fully understand the experience. They then come back to the university and discuss what they learned, typically with a faculty preceptor who serves as the referee. The goal is to engage all learners in speaking and active listening. In this model, the group does not necessarily have to make a decision, but if they do, the stakes are fairly small.

The group projects model requires students to work together in completing a term paper. For example, each student may write a paragraph, and in the final product all the paragraphs are assembled. But this is not teamwork or collaboration, Earnest said, and, generally, the students do not feel invested in the product in part because they do not believe the paper is read with sufficient attention. Furthermore, evaluating each student's contribution to the term paper is difficult.

Problem-based learning has a strong methodological foundation, but measuring the contribution of individual students is still difficult. Measuring or comparing the performance of one student team to another is difficult, as is finding problems that are amenable to this learning method and that all students embrace and are equally ready for.

Michaelson's team-based learning model had a number of valuable components, but, as with the other models, much of the student work ultimately cannot be assessed. One team's outcome can be qualitatively compared with that of another team, but an individual team's performance is not measurable.

Given the limitations of each of the models, Earnest and his colleagues devised a new model with a set of principles for what they considered optimal conditions for learning about teamwork. One condition was the requirement that the team be the unit of learning and the unit of work. With the method that Earnest and colleagues developed, the team's goal is important enough to them that they do not need a faculty preceptor. This situation more closely emulates real work environments, where there are no referees and team members need to work out challenges among themselves.

Borrowing from team- and problem-based learning models, Earnest's model has student teams receive an activity that requires group problem solving and collaboration for successful completion. Unlike the case with the group term paper, this activity cannot be easily or efficiently accomplished by single individuals or by individuals working in parallel. In addition, the team performance is measurable so that at the end of the learning activity, members can compare how they did in a standardized objective way and find out how well their team performed compared to other teams. Those teams with better collaboration receive higher scores.

In this model, an activity begins with roughly eight teams gathering in a room with a single facilitator who keeps time and directs the learning experience. The teams work in parallel to solve a multidimensional clinical puzzle in which they identify potential harms and process errors. Teams are given an hour to complete the task. At the end of that time, their work is done, and each team receives a score that is posted at the front of the room. This is followed by a debriefing that focuses on what each team did to accomplish the activity and how the team got to its answer.

Through this team-based, competitive activity, educators at the University of Colorado hope to create a language and a set of experiences that students can translate into clinical settings that will provide them with a richer and more sophisticated understanding of how to collaborate effectively.

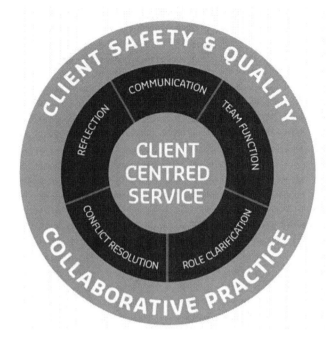

FIGURE 4-1 Interprofessional education capability framework—and the ICAT.
SOURCE: Brewer and Jones, in press.

University of Virginia

Faculty of the University of Virginia (UVA) IPE program are also interested in longitudinal assessment of student learning, said Valentina Brashers, the UVA presenter at the workshop. Their tool, the Interprofessional Teamwork Objective Structured Clinical Examination, assesses students' pre- and post-clinical/clerkship outcomes in order to better understand student learning before and after completing four IPE simulation experiences, which are done in the same year. Students are also assessed following each individual simulation experience, she added. Using the Collaborative Behaviors Observational Assessment Tool, faculty can track student achievement of competencies corresponding to a specific simulation activity. Another assessment tool used at UVA is the Team Skills Scale. According to Brashers, this tool was developed by Hepburn and colleagues (1996) to assess self-perceived team skills in the preclinical education phase.

Brashers also said that researchers from UVA are looking into how well participants of the Continuing Interprofessional Education (CIE) Program follow through on expressed commitments to change. In this Commitment to Change model, CIE participants are asked to fill out a "commitment to change" form before leaving the premises; UVA staff follow up with each participant 3 and 6 months later to ask whether the participant made the intended change. Although the results from this activity at UVA are still pending, Brashers said, studies have shown that health providers who make such commitments are more likely to change their behavior than those who do not make the commitments (Wakefield et al., 2003; Fjortoft, 2007).

University of Missouri

The University of Missouri's IPE presenter, Carla Dyer, reported how a measure of safety—decreasing hospital patient falls—has been used as the endpoint for assessing student-based interprofessional interventions in an attempt to link IPE to patient outcomes. Using patient interviews to assess student success, the research group found that despite the lack of evidence demonstrating a significant impact on patient falls—which may have been an artifact of the small sample size—93 percent of patients reported that the students' interventions had value. Furthermore, through pre- and post-intervention testing of the participating medical and nursing students, faculty did find that the students had significantly greater confidence in assessing and intervening at-risk patients after participating in the interventions.

Department of Veterans Affairs Administration

One of the evaluation tools used by the Department of Veterans Affairs (VA), reported on by Kathryn Rugen at the workshop, is the VA Learner Perception Survey. According to Rugen, this tool was modified specifically for use in primary care to include attributes of the PACT (Patient Aligned Care Teams) model of patient-centered, team-based interprofessional care. This revised survey was piloted in 2012. Rugen said that preliminary analysis showed that the trainees within the centers of excellence were reporting higher satisfaction rates, although further assessments (which are forthcoming) are needed to confirm these preliminary results.

Linköping University

At Linköping University in Sweden, Margaretha Wilhelmsson and colleagues were interested in knowing whether certain personal attributes indicated a readiness for interprofessional learning. According to Wilhelmsson, who represented the university's IPE program at the workshop, they studied approximately 700 medical and nursing students from programs across

Sweden. Using the Readiness for Interprofessional Learning instrument, they found that women and those enrolled in nursing programs displayed earlier readiness for interprofessional learning. The study included only nursing and medical students, but it does indicate that some students may be more ready than others to work collaboratively. Such increased readiness could lead to greater success in interprofessional education and collaborations (Wilhelmsson et al., 2011).

EVALUATING IPE TO INTERPROFESSIONAL PRACTICE

In her summary remarks Forum member Gillian Barclay from the Aetna Foundation said that activities are under way to measure "care coordination" in the United States. For example, she pointed out that in 2010 the National Quality Forum published *Preferred Practices and Performance Measures for Measuring and Reporting Care Coordination* (NQF, 2010), and that same year the Agency for Healthcare Research and Quality produced *Care Coordination Measures Atlas* (AHRQ, 2012). The following year the National Committee for Quality Assurance made the Care Coordination Process Measures available in addition to similar measurement publications already available from other organizations. Despite these laudable efforts to measure care coordination activities, however, no organizations are attempting to measure linkages between IPE and interprofessional practice (IPP). As Barclay said, "It is a bit disturbing because the assumption is made that care can be coordinated without really figuring out if people have competencies and skills to work together as a team. It is not as simple as just putting people there and having them coordinate care." In addition, she added, many of the indicators used to measure outcomes in care coordination come from the clinical environment, such as the 30-day readmission rate and the time spent in a waiting room. Barclay then challenged the audience to go beyond the walls of the clinical environment to use IPE-to-IPP indicators that measure outcomes in population health.

Although Forum Member Brenda Zierler from the University of Washington agreed with Barclay, she added that, from a clinical perspective, there may be difficulties with linking patient outcomes to IPE training events in the simulation lab or classroom for pre-licensure students. One reason for this is that students are trained together in team-based activities and then placed in clinical sites, one student at a time. The other issue is the inability of high-functioning clinical teams to articulate team competencies to students. This issue was also raised by Matthew Wynia of the American Medical Association, who found in a study with colleagues that team members do not always see what they do as transferrable, teachable, or something that others could adopt and learn (Mitchell et al., 2012). As a result, there are potential teachers and role models of team care that go untapped because these individuals do not recognize that their activities are teachable.

Key Messages Raised by Individual Speakers

- Implementers of IPE need to be clear about the purpose of their work so researchers can confidently analyze whether or not a program is successful. (Reeves)
- Uncertainty over how to measure IPE creates obstacles to developing competency-based models and an evidence base for IPE. (Holmboe)
- A complex, multi-sourced approach to assessment and evaluation is needed to distill the meaning and value of IPE. (Earnest and Holmboe)
- Tools for assessing interprofessional learning are being developed and refined. (Brashers, Dyer, Earnest, Forman, and Rugen)

REFERENCES

AHRQ (Agency for Healthcare Research and Quality). 2012. Patient centered medical home resource center. http://www.pcmh.ahrq.gov/portal/server.pt/community/pcmh__home/1483/pcmh_defining_the_pcmh_v2 (accessed March 4, 2013).

Brewer, M., and S. Jones. In press. An interprofessional practice capability framework focusing on safe, high quality client centred health service. *Journal of Allied Health*.

Fjortoft, N. 2007. The effectiveness of commitment to change statements on improving practice behaviors following continuing pharmacy education. *American Journal of Pharmacy Education* 71(6):112.

Hepburn, K., R. A. Tsukuda and C. Fasser. 1996. Team skills scale. In G. D. Heinemann and A. M. Zeiss, eds., *Team performance in health care: Assessment and development*. New York: Kluwer Academic/Plenum Publishers.

Mitchell, P., M. Wynia, R. Golden, B. McNellis, S. Okun, C. E. Webb, V. Rohrbach, and I. von Kohorn. 2012. *Core principles and values of effective team-based care*. Discussion Paper, Institute of Medicine, Washington, DC. http://iom.edu/Global/Perspectives/2012/TeamBasedCare.aspx (accessed March 12, 2013).

NQF (National Quality Forum). 2010. *Preferred practices and performance measures for measuring and reporting care coordination: A consensus report*. Washington, DC: NQF.

Patton, M. 2011. *Developmental evaluation: Applying complexity concepts to enhance innovation and use*. New York: Guilford Press.

Pawson, R., and N. Tilley. 1997. *Realist evaluation*. London, UK: Sage.

Reeves, S., S. Lewin, S. Espin, and M. Zwarenstein. 2010. *Interprofessional teamwork for health and social care*. Oxford, UK: Wiley-Blackwell.

Wakefield, J., C. P. Herbert, M. Maclure, C. Dormuth, J. M. Wright, J. Legare, P. Brett-MacLean, and J. Premi. 2003. Commitment to change statements can predict actual change in practice. *Journal of Continuing Education in the Health Professions* 23(2):81–92.

Wilhelmsson, M., S. Ponzer, L. O. Dahlgren, T. Timpka, and T. Faresjö. 2011. Are female students in general and nursing students more ready for teamwork and interprofessional collaboration in healthcare? *BMC Medical Education* 11:15.

5

Interprofessional Education
Within the Health System

Summary: *Interprofessional education (IPE) is part of a broader system of health and education. This chapter attempts to describe how IPE fits into the continuum of these systems. Examples of IPE that span education and practice are provided from the Department of Veterans Affairs (VA), the University of Virginia (UVA), and Kaiser Permanente. These examples led participants to question whether there are high-functioning collaborative practices that do not currently engage students but that could be opportunities for learners to better understand the values around high-functioning teams and collaborations. Vermont's Blueprint for Health was one example of such an opportunity that is described in this chapter. Following this description, there is a discussion of important health care issues involving workforce development and the expansion of the ethnic and cultural diversity of health providers and workers through IPE. The chapter closes with a discussion on the effective use of funds in IPE and in health care to lower costs while improving the value and the quality of care for patients and their caretakers, who are at the center of the health care system.*

In her role as co-chair of the workshop, Forum member Lucinda Maine of the American Association of Colleges and Pharmacy described the model for continuous improvement in clinical education and practice that was developed by the Forum and planning committee member Malcolm Cox, from the VA (see Figure 5-1). In this model, in which educational reform and interprofessional practice (IPP) are inextricably linked, the patient is at

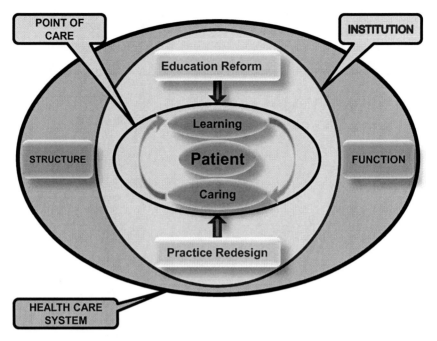

FIGURE 5-1 Patient-centered model for continuous improvement in clinical education and practice.
SOURCE: VA, 2012 (courtesy of Malcolm Cox).

the center of a clinical microsystem ("point of care") surrounded by a positively reinforcing learning and caring feedback loop. The model illustrates the fact that, collectively, many such microsystems of clinical care and education are embedded in health care systems ("institutions"). According to Cox, education reform and practice redesign are continuously interacting, so that changes in one—by way of the learning and caring feedback loop—will inevitably influence the other. Cox explained that each institutional mesosystem is, in turn, embedded in the overall health care macrosystem ("health care system"). And at each level of this complex adaptive system, myriad processes are subject to analysis and improvement.

This networked system of education and practice was the focus of many presenters at the workshop. One such presenter was Kathryn Rugen from the VA, who reported that the goal of the VA's centers of excellence in primary care education is to develop and test innovative structural and curriculum models that foster the transformation of health care training from the professional silos to interprofessional team-based education and clinical care delivery.

She said that the VA has been providing interprofessional team-based care for decades in areas such as geriatrics and palliative care but have not officially declared it as such. Because the VA has the largest medical education and health professionals training program in the United States, academic leaders there recognized the opportunity this creates for IPE. They decided to name their previously undefined model of interprofessional team-based geriatric and palliative care, and expand it to primary care training. According to Rugen, this led to what are now known as the VA centers of excellence in primary care education. The core requirements for these centers include co-direction by a physician and a nurse practitioner; joint sponsorship and engagement with academic affiliates; integrated, interprofessional teams in the workplace; and a commitment from trainees that 30 percent of their academic clinical training will be at the centers of excellence. Rugen provided the following list of primary learners:

- Physician resident trainees: internal medicine PGY 1, 2, 3, chief resident; family medicine PGY1; psychiatry
- Nurse practitioner trainees: pre-master's, pre-doctorate of nursing practice, post-master's fellows
- Postdoctorate pharmacy residents
- Postdoctorate psychology fellows and psychology interns

Besides these primary learners, there is also some engagement from the social work and nutrition areas, bachelor's degree nursing students, medical students, podiatry, and physician assistants.

Rugen said that each center balances formal IPE instruction with workplace learning and reflection that is both inter- and intraprofessional. Table 5-1 provides details about these educational strategies which use formal instruction within developmentally appropriate learning activities to support workplace learning and purposeful reflective practices. The table also lists, for each educational domain, examples of evaluation methods employed by the VA that measure what works, for whom, under what circumstances, and why.

Another program, described by workshop speaker Valentina Brashers from UVA, is similarly focused on the education-to-practice continuum. The program strives to provide clinically relevant IPE. According to Brashers, this education is required and fully integrated across the learning continuum and assessed longitudinally, it is associated with a commitment to rigorous research and dissemination of results, and it is intended to bridge the gaps between education, patient care, and patient outcomes.

The IPE innovators of the program, of which Brashers is one, developed what they call the Collaborative Care Best Practice Model to support the creation of their interprofessional education experiences. This model is based in clinical guidelines that address areas of need in the health system

TABLE 5-1 VA Centers of Excellence Educational Strategies and Evaluation Methods

Educational Domain	Definition	Activity Examples	Evaluation Examples
Shared decision making	Care is aligned with the values, references, and cultural perspective of the patient; curricula focus on the communication skills necessary to promote patients' self-efficacy.	• Ottawa Shared Decision Making Curriculum and Skill Three-Part Longitudinal Series—LEARN (Listen, Explain, Acknowledge, Recommend, and Negotiate) • Motivational Interviewing	• Mini-Clinical Evaluation Exercise • Decision Support Analysis Tool • Dyadic OPTION Scale • Learner Perception Survey–Primary Care
Sustained relationships	Care is designed to promote continuity of care; curricula focus on longitudinal learning relationships.	• Home visits • "Lost Opportunities" curriculum	• Modified Continuity of Care Index (MCCI) • Qualitative interviews • Learner Perception Survey–Primary Care • PACT continuity encounter
Interprofessional collaboration	Care is team-based, efficient, and coordinated; curricula focus on developing trustful, collaborative relationships.	• University of Toronto Centre for IPE • Huddle-Coaching Program	• Longitudinal semi-structured interviews • Team Development Measure • Readiness for Interprofessional Learning Scale
Performance improvement	Care is designed to optimize the health of populations; curricula focus on using the methodology of continuous improvement in redesigning care to achieve quality outcomes.	• Curriculum of Inquiry • Panel Management • All sites looking at emergency room visits	• Clinical outcomes • Quality Improvement Knowledge Application Tool (QIKAT)

SOURCE: Department of Veterans Affairs.

for improved teamwork, she said, adding that expert interprofessional panels choose the guidelines and develop cases and checklists of behaviors that are essential for adequate implementation of those guidelines. The checklists fully integrate both the profession-specific and the interprofessional skills for optimal guideline implementation. From these collaborative care best practices models, Brashers said, she and her colleagues can create not only clinically relevant interprofessional experiences, but also assessment opportunities. They call their collaborative-behavior observational assessment tools—which are used to assess students during interprofessional teamwork—OSCEs, or objectively structured clinical examinations. By creating tools and experiences with this method, Brashers said, it is possible to use the same process to adapt tools appropriately for the target learner. In this way the model used to assess undergraduate students is simpler than that used for residents and graduate nursing students, she said, whereas fellows, clinicians, and faculty receive what she called the "gold standard model" of assessment.

Brashers said that this process embeds IPE in a clinical base because the skills needed for interprofessional collaboration around a crashing sepsis patient are somewhat different from the skills necessary for appropriate interprofessional collaboration around an end-of-life discussion with a family member. Tailoring IPE in this way provides opportunities to develop interprofessional experiences and assessment tools that address specific patient populations, illness experiences, and care settings. The advantages to using this method, she said, are that it provides very specific and measurable learning objectives to work with, it integrates profession-specific skills with interprofessional learning so that students do not see a divide between what they need to know and how they need to deliver that care, and it establishes IPE as a core element of the clinical and clerkship experiences of students.

Although both UVA and the VA provide good examples of the continuum between education and practice, workshop speaker Dennis Helling from Kaiser Permanente Colorado Region drew the audience's attention to the second workshop objective: "identify and examine academic/practice partnerships that demonstrate purposeful modeling to advance team-based education and collaborative practice." After reading this objective, Helling said, "I think that statement and objective makes a huge assumption that there are critical numbers and access by universities to high-performing, interprofessional teams delivering interprofessional health care." But, he said, that is not always the case. He added that while there must be academic-based training on interprofessional education, the course work should be reinforced with real-life experiential practices. Helling spent some time explaining how he came to this opinion, a discussion that is captured in Box 5-1 along with a description of some of Helling's work exposing pharmacy students to high-functioning teams at Kaiser Permanente.

BOX 5-1
Dennis Helling, Pharm.D., D.Sc., FCCP, FASHP
Kaiser Permanente Colorado Region, Department of Pharmacy

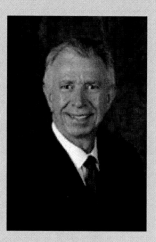

During the first 19 years of his career, Dennis Helling was an academic chair for clinical pharmacy and an associate dean for clinical affairs at the University of Iowa and then at the Texas Medical Center. He was very active in building academic programs to locate in what he hoped would be collaborative IPP sites. Often Helling felt stressed when attempting to find strong IPP sites that mirrored the principles and values he taught in the classroom about IPP. When he put the students in sites that provided sub-optimal interprofessional experiences, sometimes what he told the students in class did match up with what they found in the practice environment. It was then that Helling made a personal career decision to, as he said, "walk the talk."

IPE for Workforce Development

Sarita Verma and Maria Tassone are co-leads of the Canadian Interprofessional Health Leadership Collaborative, which is described in Appendix C. They explained the origins of IPE in Canada, which was engineered specifically to meet the health care needs of Canada. Verma began by saying that, starting in 2002, the famous Romanow commission recommended that educational programs be changed to focus on more integrated, team-

Helling left full-time academia and joined Kaiser Permanente in Denver, Colorado, 20 years ago to focus on building an advanced collaborative practice for pharmacists. In testing this collaborative practice model—on how pharmacists, physicians, nurses, and others could deliver superior care together while Pharmacy Doctorate students, residents, and fellows actively participate—Helling demonstrated the positive return on investment of pharmacy services through a rigorous evaluation of the model.

Helling said that the department where he works includes roughly 500 pharmacists and is the largest employer of pharmacists in the state of Colorado. Furthermore, he said, his institution is the largest provider of advanced practice experiences in the state of Colorado, working both with the University of Colorado and Regis University. Helling spoke with representatives from both of these universities to consider what an ideal rotation or advanced practice experience would look like. Based on these discussions, Helling determined that, ideally, the IPE experiences would increase the students' self-directed learning, their independence, and their self-confidence. They would also provide benefits to the preceptor site that would exceed the cost of the precepting. In essence, Helling said, "we would add value to the organization and to our patients." And, he added, he and his colleagues would prepare students so they were "team ready" after they finished their advanced practice experience at Kaiser.

Helling next described having students placed in each of 27 areas, including applied pharmacogenomics, travel clinics, neurology, oncology, behavioral health, geriatrics, and endocrinology. According to Helling, his department can offer opportunities to students in each of the practice sites that have clinical pharmacy specialists because the medical group and pharmacy came to an agreement that the medical group needed clinical pharmacy services to advance access, quality, and affordability.

In summarizing his talk, Helling said that he and his colleagues feel that (1) students can be trusted to work independently with supervision, (2) having an opportunity to make an impact is important, (3) students help preceptors expand their capacity and ability, and (4) an organized service program that is built on a strong, IPP prepares students to be team ready.

based approaches to meet the health care and service delivery needs of the Canadian population. The Accord on Health Care Renewal, which focuses on accessibility, quality, and affordability of care, is one agreement between the provinces and the federal government that deals with IPE.

In the mid-2000s, Verma said, an advisory committee of high-level political leaders and deputy ministers was formed that drove innovations in health care in the Canada's 13 provinces and territories. But the seminal moment for IPE was in 2004 when Health Canada provided funding for projects that launched the activities that led to health professions education reform in Canada.

Continuing the presentation, Tassone reported that IPE for collaborative patient-centered care projects originally received more than 20 million Canadian dollars over the 4 years from 2004 to 2008 to catalyze this work and to strengthen these linkages. What happened, according to Tassone, is that the early projects, about 20 of them, created the country's national exemplars in the three following areas:

1. Educational and instructional curricular activities and IPE courses,
2. Continuing professional development focusing on enhancing collaborative competencies, and
3. IPP-based learning experiences.

The first area, Tassone said, centers on curriculum activities that provide students opportunities to engage in a longitudinal curriculum. The second area incorporates a professional development perspective. A number of programs across the country started by training educators in how they can teach and model collaboration. Tassone said that those programs are increasingly being extended in order to partner with collaborations in the practice environment. There are now roughly equal numbers of educators, practitioners, and practice leaders learning these competencies, which not only relate to how they are teaching students but also to how they are behaving in practice settings. Tassone said she believes that the third area of focus resonates most with the students. This area involves IPP-based learning and includes structured experiences in which students come together to work on quality-improvement projects within a hospital or in a community setting. As an example of this experiential learning, Tassone pointed to the health mentor programs offered across the country that allow students to shadow patients with chronic diseases.

Tassone also commented on another important piece of work involving an organization that was funded and promoted by Health Canada, the Canadian Interprofessional Health Collaborative. This is a voluntary organization with a very small secretariat that provides Canadians with an opportunity to collect and distill some of the local examples and IPE innovations across Canada while also looking at work that is happening beyond the Canadian borders.

In her closing remarks, Tassone said that she thinks IPE is "a common theme across all of the professions and it's an enabler of all the things that are really important to us in health education and health care quality, safety, and sustainability of the health care system."

Similar to Tassone and Verma, Sanjay Zodpey is a Forum member heading the Forum's Innovation Collaborative. His Collaborative is out of the Public Health Foundation of India in New Delhi that is designed to build the capacity of health professionals in India by establishing a cluster for health workforce planners with a focus on the education of health professionals. One objective of their work is to identify the interdisciplinary health care leadership competencies relevant to medical, nursing, and public health professional education in India. Once these competencies are identified, Zodpey said, his collaborative plans to develop and pilot an interprofessional training model for physicians, nurses, and public health professionals to develop the leadership skills relevant to the 21st-century health systems in India.

In Uganda, workshop speaker and Innovation Collaborative lead Nelson Sewankambo worked with colleagues to introduce IPE in 2001 because there was a shortage of teachers and health workers in the country. In designing the IPE curriculum for Makerere University, Sewankambo worked closely with the Ministry of Health to ensure that its graduates entered the workforce with the right set of skills to affect the entire population and community they are trying to serve. A description of the Indian and the Ugandan innovation collaborations and how their collaborative work relates to the Global Forum can be found in Appendix C.

IPE and the Industrialization of Health Care

Workshop speaker Rosemary Gibson from the *Archives of Internal Medicine* suggested that the challenges facing IPE are related to the broader health care system in which it is operating. Considering the impact of the system on IPE, she addressed what she refers to as the "industrialization of health care," which has led to a system that values health as a commodity. She noted that within this culture patients stand a high risk of diminished safety and care.

Before providing comments on system issues related to IPE, she shared her experience of mainstreaming palliative care into the health care system as an example of a promising interprofessional enterprise. In 1995, a major study showed how poorly the U.S. health care system takes care of people at the end of life (SUPPORT Investigators, 1995). In response, the Robert Wood Johnson Foundation, where Gibson was working, made $250 million in investments to address end-of-life issues. Palliative care teams were assembled in a number of hospitals with these funds that consisted of physicians, nurses, pharmacists, clergy, and volunteers working together to care for seriously ill patients at the end of their lives. The palliative care model developed in this effort has been considered a success by those working in palliative care, with 1,500 hospitals employing palliative care teams in 2012. Furthermore, the American Academy of Hospice and Palliative

Medicine now holds its meetings jointly with hospice and palliative nurses, which Gibson called a giant leap forward.

Fifteen years after development of the palliative care teams model, Gibson said that while improvements in care have been made, what has been accomplished is putting "palliative care teams out there in rowboats to rescue people from the rising waters of the medical–industrial complex, but they are not able to stop those rising waters." As other speakers had mentioned, culture affects IPE, and the culture of the industrialization of health care definitely impacts care of patients.

Gibson made a few observations about that industrialized health care system and what it means for IPE and team-based care. She suggested that although more drugs and devices are being pushed into the system, conversation is being driven out, particularly in the inpatient setting. The system is minimizing time to talk to patients. However, the palliative care teams are an exception, and some lessons can be learned from models that have been able to work within the industrialized health care system. Gibson also suggested that such a system operates with high volume and overtreatment and is continuously being pushed to operate faster. "I'm sure you all saw the study of burnout among 46 percent of physicians, particularly emergency room physicians and internal medicine doctors," she said, referring to a 2012 study by Schattner. "The ones that did not report as much burnout were those taking care of people at the end of life." Gibson suggested that such burnout is a result of the industrialization of the health care system.

Considering the characteristics of the industrialized health care system, Gibson asked how IPE and teams can be designed to survive and thrive in this system. How will a team's function be communicated to patients in terms of accountability and individual identity within the team? Gibson suggested that the development of highly functioning teams will depend on the quality of the system in which these teams perform. As teams are being set up, efforts need to be made to create a system in which teams can function and thrive. She thinks this can be and is being done; however, an understanding of the parameters is needed within which the teams can work productively. Her suggestions were to "create those teams, make them work, but protect them and create these boundaries around them so they are preserved, so they can function, and do as they're supposed to do, while at the same time we figure out about this bigger picture, big industrial health care issues that I think we're all facing."

Collaborative Practices for IPE Experiences

The presentation by Dennis Helling led Forum and planning committee member George Thibault to ask whether some health professions other than pharmacy might take advantage of the strong collaborative environment set up by Kaiser Permanente. Although the question was posed to Helling, it was also relevant to other speakers, such as Craig Jones, who presented an excellent example of a collaborative practice during the workshop. This example, described in Box 5-2, is the Vermont Blueprint for Health, where Jones is the executive director. Another example of a practice environment that could be used for interprofessional education came from David Collier, who directs the East Carolina University Pediatric Healthy Weight Research and Treatment Center. Given that obesity is a complex bio-psycho-social disease, Collier said, the best treatment and prevention modalities are those that are interprofessional. According to Collier, obesity research and treatment offers an excellent environment for IPE. Collier said that his clinic seeks to bring many services together so that patients can see all the services at the same time; then the different health professionals work together to develop a plan that best fits the needs of a patient and his or her family. The professional expertise represented in the clinic includes pharmacy, physical therapy, nutrition, public health, periodontics, psychological and behavioral counseling, medicine, and nursing.

David Krol of the Robert Wood Johnson Foundation, who represented the foundation at the workshop, saw Collier's work as an opportunity not just to expose students to team-based care of pediatric obesity, but also to give students the chance to engage in advocacy on issues of community policy, such as the issue of vending machines in schools. Collier agreed with Krol on the importance of student engagement in community efforts against obesity. He said that his team does mentor students and facilitate student-run activities in nutrition education and physical activity promotion in communities. However, he added, sustaining the student-initiated programs is one challenge he has not yet overcome.

Forum member Gillian Barclay from the Aetna Foundation, a member of the reflection panel addressing principles and gaps in IPE, reminded the workshop participants of the Community-Oriented Primary Care movement which dated back to the 1970s and 1980s. This movement, she said, was intended to improve community health by employing principles from public health, epidemiology, and primary care (IOM, 1983; Longlett et al., 2001). A number of attempts were made during this movement to have the community intersect with academia. Barclay suggested that the lessons learned from those strategies and experiences would be extremely relevant to IPE. She then challenged the audience to think beyond the walls of the clinical environment. How, she asked, might IPE be part of population and community health in a way that could integrate health and wellness with community-based social support services? Barclay talked about the difference it would make to students' educational experiences if they were exposed to interprofessional care coordination in community settings that intersect with primary care.

BOX 5-2
Craig Jones, M.D.
Vermont Blueprint for Health

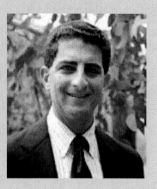

Craig Jones is the executive director of Vermont's Blueprint for Health, which is one of the state-led initiatives seeking to transform health care delivery through-out Vermont. By acting as an agent of change, Jones said, Blueprint for Health is creating a comprehensive community system of health from the current system, which contains multiple providers, practices, and insurers (Department of Vermont Health Access, 2012).

One method that Blueprint for Health is using to achieve this goal is encour-aging practices to become patient-centered medical homes (PCMHs), also known as advanced primary care practices. Jones described the National Committee for Quality Assurance's established standards and criteria for practices seeking to become patient-centered medical homes and the Blueprint for Health's role in developing a formal method of helping practices in Vermont prepare to be scored

Having funded some of this work when she was at the W.K. Kellogg Foundation, Barclay was able to speak to the workshop participants about the difficulties faculty members faced in engaging communities, especially members of the medical faculty who wanted to work with faculty members from other disciplines to focus on community needs. "It really affected their tenure or their ability to achieve tenure," she said, because such collabora-tive work may not lead to the sorts of papers and publications that could advance academic careers.

against these standards. After a practice has prepared, it is scored by an independent team from the University of Vermont; the scoring is done by a different team in order to maintain objectivity because the payment that the practice will eventually receive from insurers is based on this score. With the multi-insurer payment reforms, Jones said, all insurers share the costs and make a per-person, per-month payment that is directly proportional to the score received; thus, this additional payment represents a quality payment on top of the fee for services.

Blueprint for Health has gone to even greater measures to provide coordinated support to the citizens of Vermont, Jones said. A PCMH could be improving access, communication, and guideline-based care, he explained, but still lack the true multidisciplinary support that people need. To supplement the PCMH, Blueprint for Health asked insurers to support community health teams. These locally designed, locally organized, and integrated multidisciplinary teams work to bridge the gap of support for the general population. Although case management traditionally has been available for those with specific conditions and those who are very sick, Jones said, there was a lack of interprofessional and multidisciplinary support for the general population that the community health teams seek to fill.

Jones said that some insurers have added more professionals specialized in case management among high-risk populations to their community health teams. For example, Medicare now pays for support and service at home (SASH) teams, which are coordinators that work at the household level in publicly subsidized housing in especially high-risk Medicare populations. These SASH teams, Jones said, provide in-home supports, helping with daily activities, safety, and assessment, and then link back with the community health teams to streamline care.

Jones said that the work of the Vermont Blueprint for Health is founded on trust. Although it took time for Blueprint for Health to build the trust of those they serve, part of that trust was developed through the community teams which hired health educators who live and work within the communities they serve. Jones said that this is critically important for gaining the trust of the patients being served.

IPE for Diversity Opportunities

Gillian Barclay suggested to audience members that, when educating students in interprofessional environments, they consider those opportunities that go beyond health care and that could contribute to reducing racial and ethnic inequities in health. For example, when Jack Geiger was working in rural Mississippi in the 1960s, he saw the built environment as a contributor to poor patient outcomes, so he created an IPP that involved those sectors in the built environment that could help improve nutrition. Aetna Foundation is funding some of the evaluation measures within this unique IPP to see how the farmers and farmers markets, physicians, managers, and chief executive officers of these community health centers develop an interprofessional process to improve the health outcomes of patients and their communities. According to Barclay, this is the sort of culture shift to which students should be exposed. However, it is not enough to get students from different professions together; it is also important to pay close attention to race and ethnicity, looking closely at community needs and building the interprofessional training on those needs.

Melissa Simon from Northwestern University, who participated in the workshop, emphasized the opportunity that IPE brings for increasing diversity not just in professions, but also in race, religious background, sexual orientation, and other factors. This discussion resonated with the Forum member Beverly Malone, who pointed out that the main diversity issue being discussed at the workshop was differences among professional groups. Adding a consideration of color, race, and underrepresented groups, she said, makes the conversation much more complex. Although Malone said she was not sure how to weave the complex issues of diversity into the discussions and the fabric of interprofessional education, she said she felt strongly that members of the Forum need to address such issues before it is too late.

Health Disparities

The United States spends more per capita on health care than any other developed nation, yet, in comparison, Americans have shorter lives and poorer health, according to a recent report by the Institute of Medicine (2013). In looking at the U.S. health care spending curve (see Figure 5-2), small-group leader Thomas Feeley of the MD Anderson Cancer Center pointed out that U.S. spending on health care rose rapidly from the 1960s to today, when it is a total of $2.8 trillion, and that U.S. spending is projected to increase even further, to $4.6 trillion, by 2020. The United States now spends more than $8,000 per person on health, which is double the spending of the United Kingdom and Canada and more than 60 times that of any African nation (OECD, 2012). However, as was pointed out by workshop speaker Paul Worley from the School of Medicine at Flinders University, Australia, what is lost in these statistics is that spending on health is not uniform in developed countries. In his presentation, Worley cited the work of Michael Marmot (2005), which notes that there are socioeconomic disparities in health outcomes even within the richest cities of the world. A disparity in spending and in health outcomes has also been reported in the United States (Bustamante and Chen, 2011), although poor health outcomes may not result only from disparities in health care spending (Lê Cook and Manning, 2009).

Forum and planning committee member Jan De Maeseneer from

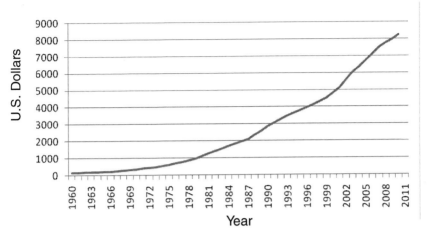

FIGURE 5-2 Mean per capita expenditure on health in the United States: 1960–2011.
SOURCE: OECD, 2012.

Ghent University in Belgium made an important point concerning the situation in sub-Saharan Africa, which is quite different from that of the United States. The Abuja Declaration of 2001 committed governments to spending at least 15 percent of their annual budgets on improvements to the health sector, De Maeseneer noted. However, on average, southern African nations today spend less than 3 percent of gross domestic product on health (World Bank, 2011). Given this stark contrast, Feeley—who led the breakout group on cost—and De Maeseneer agreed that it is appropriate to reframe the focus to reducing health care costs in areas where spending is excessive and that increased spending on health should be the focus of underserved populations. De Maeseneer and Feeley suggested reframing the discussion in terms of improving the "value" of health care. In this way, there is a balance between costs and outcomes, so an ideal health care system improves value when it improves outcomes without increasing cost. When costs are reduced, Feeley said, the reduction does not impair outcomes; such outcomes focus on the patient or the person and take into account what patients think are important outcomes in their care.

Effective Use of Funds in IPE and Health Care

Paul Grundy, who is the director of healthcare transformation at IBM, offered the perspective of an employer of health professional graduates. IBM is the largest corporate employer in Vermont, he said, and having worked closely with both a Republican and a Democratic governor, Grundy said he and his colleagues at IBM understand that a healthy workforce exists only within a healthy community. As a result of IBM's holistic care, he said, the company's trend line is down 11 percent, while trend lines are up 36 percent across the country. He attributed this success to IBM's effective, team-based, person-centered care. For example, when an IBM employee is diagnosed with diabetes, a care-coordinator from the employee's medical home exercises with the employee and educates him or her on proper food selection at local supermarket. Although the example Grundy pointed to was in Vermont, he was quick to add that similar care teams have been established in other states, such as Minnesota and North Carolina. These PCMHs were started by IBM and other organizations in 2006, and, as Grundy emphasized, this model is premised on greater access to primary care leading to healthier populations and decreased spending on costly treatments. The approach is team-based and patient-centered, and, according to the Agency for Healthcare Research and Quality, the team of providers cares for all of a patient's physical and mental health care needs from prevention and wellness through chronic care (AHRQ, 2012). At the close of his presentation, Grundy strongly encouraged educators to expose health professions students to cost-effective, collaborative care models like the PCMHs so that job applicants will be ready to begin work as a team and will not require 3 to 4 years of retraining to get them to become effective collaborators and team members. Also, he said, learning from cost-effective collaborative care models will help break the cycle of overspending that wastes billions of dollars every year in the United States (IOM, 2013).

Forum co-chair Afaf Meleis of the University of Pennsylvania School of Nursing questioned speakers who use IPE as an educational innovation to see whether they found IPE in education or team work in health care to be a financial burden or a cost savings. She also asked if there are ways by which educators and health professionals could deliver quality of care and IPE education economically.

Workshop speaker Elizabeth Speakman from Thomas Jefferson University began her response to Meleis's question with an example. She said that at some point the deans at her institution complained that faculty were spending large amounts of time with IPE. As a result, Speakman said, her institution now takes full advantage of existing IPE experiences such as the Disposition Dilemma in Rehabilitation Medicine and team-based rounds in surgery. By bringing the student to what is already taking place, Speakman said, the work is more cost-effective than bringing a new team together and having the faculty spend time developing the experience.

Workshop speaker Carla Dyer from the University of Missouri agreed with Speakman and added that when she and her colleagues work on their Achieving Competence Today program with their integrated residents, they ask department chairs which faculty members might be available for IPE training. They often stress a preference for faculty members who are new to the institution or who are early faculty who are in need of some quality improvement education. According to Dyer, a chair is asked to give protected time for the roughly 8 hours required for training over the course of 3 months. In return for this investment, the faculty members develop relationships with new types of health professional students and obtain an additional skill set that can be applied to their own clinical setting. Thus, Dyer said, everybody benefits.

The third speaker in the session, Dennis Helling, also emphasized the need for the work to be a "win-win" in terms of finances. He commented on the tension that exists between very active practice sites and academic institutions wanting to put students there. Creating and maintaining a learning environment in a practice setting takes time that can slow the pace of a busy team. It also takes a lot of time to coordinate all the students, and this draws preceptors away from other work. In making the student experience cost effective and thus justify the time spent preparing the experience, Helling explained that sometimes students pay for the advanced practice experience; other times funding is used that supports residents, research fellows, or a joint faculty position in their unit. Financial support and time are very real issues when delivering large numbers of advanced practice experiences said Helling.

In his report back to the participants about the breakout group discussions he had led on lower cost, Thomas Feeley talked about the "value proposition" in health care. This refers to a balance between health outcomes and dollars expended, and those outcomes need to be patient-centered outcomes. He advised educators and health providers to better understand what the patients think are important outcomes in their care, and then he described the framework change that he proposed to focus on for improving outcomes and quality while decreasing cost.

Feeley continued his report by describing his group's discussions based on the five areas of innovation noted in first objective of the breakout group session: curricular innovations, pedagogic innovations, cultural elements, human resources for health, and metrics. In the case of curricular design, Feeley said, health economics and quality improvement could be taught more broadly. The curriculum might also provide better critical and systems thinking, better communication skills, and better information and knowledge about information technology.

For pedagogic innovations, Feeley felt that simulation has tremendous appeal. There are some barriers, such as finding experienced staff, creating realistic scenarios, and general acceptance by educators, but regardless of the barriers, he said, simulation is generally thought to be an extremely important tool for interprofessional education. Another pedagogic innovation Feeley noted was the greater engagement of nonacademic health care schools, a step that could be cost-effective. The partners might include community colleges and various nontraditional partners that could influence IPE with their unique perspectives, leading to breakthrough innovations. Feeley said that such innovative ideas are appearing already with social media, gaming, and engineering. One other possible pedagogic innovation would be for interprofessional grand rounds to receive a greater focus than the traditional siloed grand rounds.

In the area of culture, Feeley said there appears to be a disconnect between what educators view as needed in the health care workforce and what providers feel they need. Feeley identified learning opportunities to build the workforce from such things as task sharing and by applying experiences from the military, which has always focused on cost-effective, high-quality care. Feeley was quick to point out that task sharing is distinct from task shifting, which is very important in the cost discussion. Almost every time there is a cost discussion in the United States, it involves who can do the best job at the lowest cost, he said, but the responsibility for high quality is not shifted from one to another. Quality is a responsibility that needs to be "shared" among all health workers, regardless of the remuneration provided for accomplishing the task. Adding to the human resources comments, Feeley asked how people other than health professionals, such as patients, caregivers, volunteers, aides, and clerks, can be included in the conversations about what is needed to provide high-quality, lower-cost health and health care.

Parenthetically, Feeley said, patients in the United States are not engaged in the cost of their care, and that is a huge problem. It is equally important to find better definitions of cost and of whose cost is being described—the provider, the payer, government, or the patient. This leads to the notion of metrics. According to Feeley, measurements are often described in terms of money or dollars, but metrics could also include human values that are important to patients. Also, he said that data systems, which are critical for measurement, are incredibly deficient.

There is much energy and optimism, Feeley said, but not much proof that IPE improves values or that it is the right starting point in health care. Obtaining such proof may require rethinking who is on the team (i.e., patients, caretakers, etc.) and how health care is structured. Given that prevention and early detection will lower costs, Feeley said, how might a system transition from health care to one that ensures better health?

In closing, Feeley acknowledged that many provider organizations and many governments are looking at controlling costs. He also encouraged providers and educators to better educate the public about health costs. "It is safe to talk about costs," said Feeley, "and we need to all address how we do more with less."

> ### Key Messages Raised by Individual Speakers
>
> - Education reform and practice redesign are continuously interacting. (Brashers, Cox, Helling, and Rugen)
> - Course work in IPE must be reinforced with real-life experiential practices. (Brashers, Helling, Rugen, Sewankambo, Tassone, and Verma)
> - IPE could be part of a population and community health system that could integrate health and wellness with community-based social support services. (Barclay and Feeley)
> - IPE brings opportunities for expanding diversity not just in professions but also in race, religious background, and sexual orientation. (Malone and Simon)
> - An ideal health care system improves value when it improves outcomes without increasing cost. (De Maeseneer and Feeley)

REFERENCES

AHRQ (Agency for Healthcare Research and Quality). 2012. *Patient centered medical home resource center.* http://www.pcmh.ahrq.gov/portal/server.pt/community/pcmh__ home/1483/pcmh_defining_the_pcmh_v2 (accessed March 4, 2013).

Bustamante, A. V., and J. Chen. 2011. Physicians cite hurdles ranging from lack of coverage to poor communication in providing high-quality care to Latinos. *Health Affairs* 30(10): 1921–1929.

Department of Vermont Health Access. 2012. *Vermont Blueprint for Health 2011 annual report.* Williston, VT: Department of Vermont Health Access.

IOM (Institute of Medicine). 1983. *Community oriented primary care: New directions for health services delivery.* Washington, DC: National Academy Press.

IOM. 2013. *Best care at lower cost: The path to continuously learning health care in America.* Washington, DC: The National Academies Press.

Lê Cook, B., and W. Manning. 2009. Measuring racial/ethnic disparities across the distribution of health care expenditures. *Health Services Research* 44(5, Pt. 1):1603–1621.

Longlett, S. K., J. E. Kruse, and R. M. Wesley. 2001. Community-oriented primary care: Critical assessment and implications for resident education. *Journal of the American Board of Family Practice* 14(2):141–147.

Marmot, M. 2005. Social determinants of health inequalities. *Lancet* 365:1099–1104.

OECD (Organisation for Economic Co-operation and Development). *OECD health data 2012—frequently requested data.* http://www.oecd.org/els/health-systems/oecdhealth data2012-frequentlyrequesteddata.htm (accessed March 4, 2013).

Schattner, E. 2012. The physician burnout epidemic: What it means for patients and reform. *The Atlantic.* http://www.theatlantic.com/health/archive/2012/08/the-physician-burnout-epidemic-what-it-means-for-patients-and-reform/261418 (accessed March 4, 2013).

SUPPORT Investigators. 1995. A controlled trial to improve care for seriously ill hospitalized patients. *JAMA* 274(20):8.

World Bank. 2011. *Global economic perspectives regional annex: Sub-Saharan Africa.* http:// siteresources.worldbank.org/INTGEP/Resources/335315-1307471336123/7983902-1307479336019/AFR-Annex.pdf (accessed March 4, 2013).

6

Learning from Students, Patients, and Communities

Summary: *In this chapter, students who have learned or are currently learning through interprofessional environments express their opinions on what they believe the educators did right in interprofessional education (IPE) and where IPE could possibly be strengthened. The description of the students' views of IPE is followed by a description of Sally Okun's presentation at the workshop. Okun spoke about the benefits of involving patients, caretakers, and communities in team-based and collaborative practices and about how patients can assist in IPE if given the information they need to understand its value. A key message from Okun's presentation was to get to the "real place" by listening to patients and caretakers, then learn from them and work with them. A similar message was offered by students and the presenter Paul Worley, who encouraged educators to provide students with real-life opportunities that could transform their lives.*

STUDENT EXPERIENCES AND TRANSFORMATIONS

In his closing address at the workshop, Paul Worley from the School of Medicine at Flinders University, Australia, described what he heard workshop participants repeatedly describe as a "transformation of the health care system." However, Worley suggested, the transformation of a system starts with people or, more specifically, with individuals. He encouraged the audience to listen to students and to encourage that transformation to occur in their students. It is through the power of the students, Worley said, that educators will find enthusiastic promoters of social accountability and "a whole lot of other things as well." These "other things" Worley alluded to were made concrete in the example he offered about one of his students he called, "Lucy," who is described in Box 6-1.

In addition to the student Sandeep Kishore, whose comments are summarized in Chapter 2, the workshop participants also heard from a panel of four students who represented nursing, medicine, and pharmacy. The

BOX 6-1
Lucy, M.D.
Global Physician Trainee

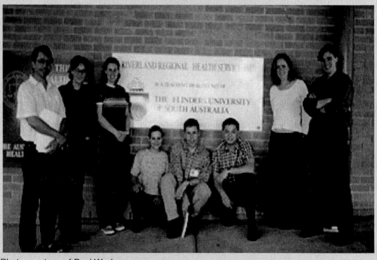

Photo courtesy of Paul Worley.

Paul Worley, dean of the School of Medicine at Flinders University in Australia, spoke about a student he knew who was transformed by her educational process. She came from a city environment and had always wanted to be a city pediatrician. Like the other medical students at Flinders, this student had the opportunity to study for an entire year in a small rural community in Australia—an opportunity that she accepted. She worked in a remote, underserved area where the need for health-related interventions and health care was immense. That experience transformed her, Worley said.

After graduation this student—whom Worley referred to as "Lucy," although that was not her real name—decided that instead of working as a pediatrician, moderator of the session, Mohammed Ali, a founding member of the Young Professionals–Chronic Disease Network based at Emory University, commented that it is not just the future employers or the supply side that has a vested interest in educating students to work collaboratively; the students themselves are seeking these opportunities. In the end, he added, it might be the students who propel educators to do more interprofessionally because it seems that students are beginning to demand an IPE to learn

she wanted global physician training. She went to work in Southern Sudan with Médecins Sans Frontières because none of the doctors who had been trained in Sudan wanted to work in this challenging area. While in South Sudan, Worley said, Lucy lived in what was called a "privileged hut" because it had a dug-out section in the hut beneath the level of the ground in which she slept. The reason it was dug out and the reason she was privileged was that when the bandits came through with their submachine guns and terrorized the village, the bullets would fly over her, rather than at her head level, as they would have if she had slept on a bed above the ground.

As Worley put it, "Some would say that just going and working there is evidence enough that there was a transformation in this person." But there was more. Lucy e-mailed him one night asking his advice as to whether she had "done the right thing." Lucy described being confronted by a patient who came to her seeking medical attention because she had been bleeding for a week post-delivery. The reason for the bleeding, which Lucy understood, was that the woman had not delivered her placenta. Lucy knew what to do technically to be able to stop the bleeding, Worley said, and she also knew that the woman needed a blood transfusion. The challenge Lucy faced was to try to find an HIV-negative, O-positive blood donor.

Worley described what Lucy did next as "the real transformation." Knowing that she herself was O positive, Lucy lay down on a mat next to her patient, put a needle into her own arm, took a liter of blood and gave that blood to the patient. In her e-mail to Worley she asked, "Did I do the right thing?" Lucy knew that if the woman did not get blood quickly, she would die no matter how good Lucy's technical skills were or how she learned them. Lucy had the head knowledge, Worley said, and she had the hand knowledge, but it was equally important that she had the heart knowledge.

Worley said that he sensed that the transformation that Lucy experienced was what many of the workshop participants were trying to convey to their students. The goal is not just to give technical skills or to transmit information or to inspire, but to change the hearts of the people who are the next generation of health professionals. Lucy did not learn what she did from a textbook or from a curriculum—she learned it from being given the space in the curriculum to get to know her patients as people. Getting to know her patients as people, Worley said, was the transformational opportunity that changed Lucy's life.

how to work more effectively together in an effort to improve patient- and person-centered care.

Angella Sandra Namwase spoke first in the session. Namwase is currently at Makerere University in Uganda pursing a degree in nursing while holding several leadership roles with the Medical Students Association and the Students Professionalism and Ethics Club in Uganda. According to Namwase, IPE helps students appreciate other professionals and helps students avoid developing negative stereotypes that could impede future work with other students. Although the size of the IPE class at Makerere can at times be overwhelming, Namwase said, she was quick to point out the advantages of shared learning. The example she offered came from her hospital rotation where the students noticed that challenges in the hospital wards that could best be addressed with assistance from the biomedical engineering students on their team. In essence, Namwase said, the main advantage of IPE is that it helps students appreciate teamwork and build an interprofessional social network while being trained as health professionals.

The social perspective of interprofessional education resonated with Erin Abu-Rish, who presented next. Abu-Rish is a second-degree nurse who said she is now pursuing a Ph.D. from the University of Washington because of the extensive opportunities for interdisciplinary research. According to Abu-Rish, social interactions outside of work time are important for students and faculty to continue learning about each other's roles. This extracurricular activity adds tremendous value to the interprofessional experience for both faculty and students, she said.

In addition to pointing out the value of extracurricular activities, Abu-Rish offered four other suggestions for IPE leaders from her perspective as a student. The advice, she said, drew on her varied IPE experiences, including dental service learning trips to a small community in Honduras, starting the Institute for Healthcare Improvement (IHI) open school chapter at the University of Washington, and publishing in the *Journal of Interprofessional Care*. One of these messages was that small group activities, problem-based learning, and interactive approaches to education draw students in and make the education more memorable. And, she added, team debriefs are effective and need to be positively oriented and well facilitated. A third suggestion was to encourage positive interactions early and often in order to develop an interprofessional culture that includes social interactions outside of class time. This has been an important part of their IPE approach with their IHI open school group where people can get to know other health professional students by name and on a personal level.

Fourth, said Abu-Rish, support for and facilitation of student involvement helps increase the sustainability of student organizations and reduces barriers to participation. She cited the example of her work with the Project Chance grant. As Abu-Rish explained it, her interprofessional team of students spent the vast majority of the funding period trying to figure out how to work together, how to engage patients, and how to obtain institutional review board approval. That is the point that students want to get to—they want to be able to work with patients together as a team. The final two thoughts Abu-Rish offered to the workshop participants were to strengthen linkages between interprofessional education and practice and to facilitate more interprofessional faculty development in order to expand the pool of faculty members who are IPE competent and willing to support innovative approaches to education.

Thomas Lewis, a first-year psychiatry resident from the Medical University of South Carolina (MUSC), was the next to speak. He discussed his interprofessional education experiences at medical school and how he applied those experiences in a clinical setting. Lewis said he first got involved with IPE through the Student Interprofessional Society (SIPS) at MUSC. SIPS is a part of the Creating Collaborative Care initiative established by his mentor, Amy Blue, several years ago. Lewis said that this program was similar to the one discussed by Erin Abu-Rish in that it focused more on the social aspect of interprofessionalism. According to Lewis, the program brought students together from different health professional schools for monthly meetings that highlighted examples of good teamwork going on at the medical university as well as in community service projects. The group provided students a chance to get to know each other as students, to talk about their different programs' strengths and weaknesses, and to compare the challenges that each was facing in his or her own professional education.

Another important educational opportunity Lewis discussed was his participation in the pilot IPE course at MUSC. The course was optional at first but is now required. In that class, he worked on root cause analyses with an interprofessional group of students; they would look at a patient's case and discuss what went wrong with the case, what could have been done differently, and where communication broke down among the different professions. That, said Lewis, was very helpful for him, especially when he started his clinical rotation as an intern and already knew how to engage with other health professionals, such as nurses, respiratory therapists, and physical therapists.

Those are examples of the way in which interprofessional education shaped his thinking, Lewis said. "I say it really helped me understand where the other professions came into play, how we can work together, and at the end of the day the common theme is patient care. It really boils down to providing good patient care and understanding our own professions to do that together."

A point brought up by Lewis in his presentation—and echoed by the next speaker, Jenny Wong, a third-year pharmacy student from the University of Minnesota—concerned the message being sent to students when interprofessional education is an optional instead of a required course. When it is required, Lewis said, it sends a clear message that it is something important that the student needs to learn. Wong agreed with that. In her education, she said, there was one required interprofessional course. But, she said, that course exposed her to IPE, which was the impetus for her pursuit of more interprofessional opportunities at the university. As she reflected upon her IPE experiences at the university, she said that she felt that the elective IPE courses helped her learn about what interprofessionalism is and that her experience at the student-run clinic helped her apply the theoretical knowledge in practice. Despite her high regard for the interprofessional opportunities afforded to her at the university, Wong would have liked a broader exposure to other health professions, such as physical therapy, dentistry, public health, and medicine; most of her interprofessional experiences were with nursing only, she said, which she found limiting.

A key observation that Wong said she made during her IPE experience was that in the rotations there is a difference between actual collaboration and a team made up of multiple different disciplines. As she put it, "I can have teammates from medicine, nutrition, and nursing, but if they do not talk to each other, then that is not IPE, and that is just a different Skittles mix of professionals."

Wong also said that she would have liked more practice-based interprofessional experiences earlier in her education. According to Wong, it was not until her third year that she had a simulation in which nursing and pharmacy students were working together that was not paper-based. It was through her academic experience and working with patients that she was able to appreciate the value of interprofessional work. As Wong explained it, it really helped her "see how this interdisciplinary system helped my patient, because now [my patient] is actually fully controlled in all three disease states because he had a continuation of care with every single one of those professions that actually came to help him."

LEARNING FROM PEOPLE

Sally Okun from PatientsLikeMe, who led the breakout group on enhanced access, provided a synopsis of that group's discussions. Her small group was asked to consider five areas of potential innovation within the general area of enhanced access; those five areas were culture, pedagogy, curriculum, metrics, and human resources for health (HRH). Okun started her report to the workshop participants by saying that one of the things her group was charged with was to think about enhanced access in terms of the education of patients and populations as learners and educators of team-based, collaborative care. She reported trying to address this charge from a global perspective of what persons and patients and populations and communities might need to understand about IPE and what it might mean to them.

To do this, her group positioned its core values within a framework that focuses on social accountability. She reported that with this structure it could become possible to determine what patients or persons would need to know about IPE and that, with this better understanding, patients could then become the teachers of health providers and the educators of students in how health professionals might better engage them and their community.

The main message Okun and her group promoted was to turn the discussions into actions by getting to the "Genba," which is a Japanese term for the real place. There are a number of resources that could be helpful in creating actionable next steps where real people with real problems are located, she said. For example, input from the community regarding its priorities and how health professional educators and providers could best meet these community-defined priorities would be helpful. Okun said that accomplishing this will involve knowing who the best person is to lead an intervention and when and where the intervention should take place. To obtain this information, Okun and her group encouraged optimizing nontraditional pathways of health care delivery and health care education in order to more fully uncover what patients and their families and people within a community think would benefit them the most. Okun emphasized the importance of community engagement for health providers and educators to better understand the selected priorities of the people in the community they serve. Without that understanding, educators may end up designing curricula in different settings that do not meet the overall needs of the people who reside in that community.

By framing IPE within a social accountability context, educators can begin to integrate a culturally diverse IPE with collaborative care models at the person, community, and population level. Involving multiple professions in one team, created with the "real place" in mind, will likely better reflects the community the team is designed to serve with regard to race and ethnicity, said Okun. This team will be made up of culturally sensitive members who are more likely to connect with and possibly build a trusting relationship with their patients and thus make positive health outcomes more probable.

In considering pedagogic innovations—or as some Forum members prefer "androgogic" innovations that targets adult teaching methods—Okun stressed that it is important to create active learning processes that enhance access to "the right people at the right time." This could include better use of technology by learners and patients of all ages and in all communities. It could also include a meaningful involvement of students by providing them access to communities and patients, which can provide a unique and memorable form of education.

For curricular innovations, Okun said that she believes feeling that the redesign of the curriculum needed to be developed after a full inventory of the resources had been conducted and after there was a firm grasp of the needs of the individuals and populations being served within the system. Educators should be integrating with patients and people within the community so that they can understand and learn from those who would be the beneficiaries of their efforts.

Like the other presenters at the workshop, Okun reported that she and her group struggled with how to measure the impact of the programs that would be designed based on her group's ideas. However, she did comment that the members of her group emphasized their desire to consider the return on investment or the impact of such community-based innovations on health at both the individual level and the population level. When these community and population impacts are understood, Okun said, it might be possible to suggest metrics that measure outcomes for patients, as measured by patients first and understood by the health professionals second. Okun added that a good social accountability metric does not yet exist, but she said that having such a tool would be useful in assessing student learning and in evaluating IPE programs.

In her comments, Okun described her group's desire to include care-givers from within the community and the population in designing IPE, explaining that the patients themselves are vulnerable because they are ill. Okun also emphasized the urgency for acting immediately if IPE innovators in the United States are to seize current opportunities through accountable care organizations, primary care, medical home models, and accreditation standards. However, Okun warned innovators to be careful not to create IPE in silos, which could then develop its own set of silos. Finally, she said, educators and health professionals need to get to the "real place" where real people with real problems are. Listen to the patients and the caretakers, she said, learn from them and work with them to identify resources and reveal redundancies that should be removed and that do not provide a return on investment. Uncover gaps in the health and educational systems, correct them, and then ultimately find ways of measuring success and of integrating the social accountability piece into that the model.

Empowering Patients

Forum member and workshop speaker Marilyn Chow from Kaiser Permanente suggested that an interesting perspective might arise if patients and their caretakers were educated and empowered to select their own team. What might this look like? One possibility, Chow said, is that patients and their families might fire a poorly functioning team. Forum member and workshop speaker Elizabeth Goldblatt from the Academic Consortium for Complementary and Alternative Health Care added that if individuals assembled their own health care teams, the makeup of a team might include both conventional and alternative health providers. She supported her comment by referring to the work of David Eisenberg and colleagues (2001, 2012), which suggests value in combining conventional care with complementary and alternative medicine. But as one participant pointed out, the public still does not know which places provide safe care. Patient advocate Rosemary Gibson from *Archives of Internal Medicine* asked, "How might patients learn to trust their providers within a team-based system?" This triggered a response from speaker Paul Grundy, the Global Director of IBM Healthcare Transformation. He said that the trust issue is why IBM has been pushing so hard for the medical home model. The most trusting relationship that exists in humanity outside of one's family is that between a patient and his or her healer, he said. IBM wants to put in place a structure that makes that trust trustworthy. As Sally Okun remarked, mechanisms need to be put in place that will help patients know they can trust and depend on the systems being built. Furthermore, educators and practitioners can learn from patients, who can be a source of data. This sort of relationship will reinforce the partnership between patients and their providers. Trust among health providers is also important, and speaker Craig Jones, the executive director of Vermont Blueprint for Health, commented that providers work within two systems of trust. The first involves trusting a new organization of care in a situation in which providers fear losing revenue and control. The second involves demonstrating an objective way of evaluating care under the new system, so that trust can be obtained through measurable outcomes. When providers realize their livelihoods are not threatened and when there is verifiable objective evidence that the concept works, Jones said, then trust evolves among providers of care and between providers and patients.

Workshop speaker Stefanus Snyman from Stellenbosch University highlighted person- and people-centered care when responding to a question about how patients reacted to receiving a more holistic clinical assessment through the World Health Organization (WHO) International Classification of Functioning, Disability and Health (ICF) framework (described in Chapter 2). He replied that patients were thrilled. They were thrilled because for the first time they felt they were being treated as persons and that health providers took into consideration all aspects of their lives. But the real value came, he said, when students and communities joined together. In the example Snyman cited, students identified a longstanding pediatric diarrhea problem in one township while conducting home visits. They then worked with parents and city officials to resolve the diarrhea in 2 days versus the months or years it usually takes to resolve such issues. By using the ICF framework, Snyman said, students were forced to take greater ownership and to find solutions to problems affecting all aspects of their patients' lives. This example shows that students are equipped to become change agents to improve patient outcomes and to strengthen health systems. And, as Paul Worley said, "The key is to give learners enough space to be the amazing creative individuals they are."

Key Messages Raised by Individual Speakers

- Students are beginning to demand an interprofessional education. (Abu-Rish, Ali, Lewis, and Wong)
- IPE helps students appreciate other professionals and avoid developing negative stereotypes. (Lewis and Namwase)
- When IPE is a required course, it sends a message to students that IPE is important. (Lewis and Wong)
- Provide interprofessional education experiences that are real and memorable and that enhance access of students to patients, caretakers, and communities. (Abu-Rish, Okun, Snyman, Wong, and Worley)
- Include caregivers from within the community and the population when designing IPE, and for understanding the needs and selected priorities of target populations. (Okun)

REFERENCES

Eisenberg, D. M., R. C. Kessler, M. I. van Rompay, T. J. Kaptchuk, S. A. Wilkey, S. Appel, and R. B. Davis. 2001. Perceptions about complementary therapies relative to conventional therapies among adults who use both: Results from a national survey. *Annals of Internal Medicine* 135(5):344–351.

Eisenberg, D. M., J. E. Buring, A. L. Hrbek, R. B. Davis, M. T. Connelly, D. C. Cherkin, D. B. Levy, M. Cunningham, B. O'Connor, and D. E. Post. 2012. A model of integrative care for low-back pain. *Journal of Alternative and Complementary Medicine* 18(4):354–362.

Frenk, J., L. Chen, Z. A. Bhutta, J. Cohen, N. Crisp, T. Evans, H. Fineberg, P. Garcia, Y. Ke, P. Kelley, B. Kistnasamy, A. Meleis, D. Naylor, A. Pablos-Mendez, S. Reddy, S. Scrimshaw, J. Sepulveda, D. Serwadda, and H. Zurayk. 2010. Health professionals for a new century: Transforming education to strengthen health systems in an interdependent world. *Lancet* 376(9756):1923–1958.

7

Moving Forward by Looking Back

Summary: *This chapter captures the presentations of several speakers who reflected upon the ideas, presentations, and discussions offered at the two workshops. Workshop speakers Madeline Schmitt and Martha Gaines provided summaries that looked into recent and distant past experiences with interprofessional education (IPE) and considered present opportunities that could lead to future innovations in IPE and collaborative practice. In particular, Schmitt and others considered how examples from the 1960s and 1970s might inform today's innovators. Barbara Brandt, the director of the new National Coordinating Center for Interprofessional Education and Collaborative Practice, is one such innovator who spoke about the center at the workshop. Her presentation is summarized here, followed by the final reflections of Martha Gaines. In her remarks, Gaines posed a series of provocative questions designed to stimulate thinking that might spark new ideas and create more innovations like those that resulted in the new National Coordinating Center.*

REFLECTIONS

Workshop I

As a workshop planning committee member who was instrumental in helping plan the first workshop, Forum member Madeline Schmitt from the University of Rochester was well positioned to reflect upon that first meeting. In her reflections Schmitt looked back at the workshop objectives to determine how well they had been addressed. Part of the first objective was "to engage in forward-looking dialogue." Schmitt said that the workshop had effectively initiated those conversations. However, in thinking back, she said she sensed some tension as participants raised known challenges and as diverse opinions were offered about how educators and health professionals might address such challenges and take advantage of current opportunities, particularly in the United States. Schmitt also said that she believed the participants embraced the second part of the first objective concerning the importance of aligning health professions education with the needs of clinical practice, consumers, and health care delivery systems.

Schmitt then read the second objective, which was "to explore the opportunity for shared decision making, distributed leadership, and team-based care amongst other interprofessional education and practice innovations to fundamentally change health professions' curricula, pedagogy, culture, human resources, and assessment and evaluation metrics." In her opinion, she said, IPE per se was not as much a part of the general discussion as it might have been. However, she said, the breakout groups more adequately focused on IPE in the five areas noted in the objective. Then Schmitt read objective three, which was "to discuss how innovations in IPE will impact patient and population health as identified by the triple aim of better health, higher quality, and lower cost." Again Schmitt said she thought that the workshop presentations and discussions did address this objective and that there were beginning conversations about how to think differently about measuring IPE and possibly reshaping the language.

Schmitt shared two points that she said might help with future workshop planning. First, would be the inclusion of a holistic, person-centered perspective. She noted that some of the workshop presenters had described useful tools that could help introduce or reintroduce this perspective into health professions education. The second would be to pay considerable attention to the many ways innovators address communities, population demands, and patient requirements within health care delivery systems when designing future workshop agendas. In this regard, Schmitt noted that one particular message—that service learning gets educators and health professionals into the community, and gets students into the community early—was touched on repeatedly throughout the workshop. But there was also the message that service learning is often disconnected from the clinical experiences that come after service learning. Judging from the Uganda experience with community-based IPE, she said, it seems to be within the third year that IPE drops off as students begin their clinical experiences. Judging from the Uganda experience with community-based IPE, she said, it seems to be within the third year that IPE drops off as students begin their clinical experiences.

Schmitt then discussed what she had heard about institutional leadership; in particular, she noted that collaborative leadership is critically important in moving the IPE agenda forward. One of the most significant insights the workshop provided to her involved the larger political, economic, and cultural context within which educators and health professionals are trying to work. For example, there were robust discussions at the workshop about moving toward social accountability as a broad framework for action. It was then that Schmitt realized the patient perspective may not be getting adequate attention, particularly in the U.S. health care system. The U.S. health care system is benefitting financially from business models—including the business models of publicly traded health care corporations—that often are unfamiliar to many health educators, researchers, and IPE innovators. The United States is now seeing the ultimate consequences of the economic and corporate imperative which neglects social accountability, Schmitt said, noting that the United States does have sufficient levels of primary care. After acknowledging comments from non-U.S. workshop participants who called primary care an "imperative," Schmitt said that addressing this issue is not a simple process. She reflected on the United States in the 1960s and 1970s, when there also was a huge need for primary care, but, despite the need, neither a robust primary care system nor interprofessional education became a priority.

Before Schmitt's presentation, another workshop speaker had reminded the audience about the Declaration of Alma Ata (WHO, 1978). This was an attempt in 1978 to bring together health leadership from around the world to promote expansion of primary care and to propose what was called "health for all." This document emphasized that health is more than simply the absence of disease; it also includes the most positive aspects of mental, physical, and environmental health (WHO, 1981). Although the expansion of primary health was certainly a laudable goal, as the participant pointed out, those who tried to move "health for all" concepts forward came to realize just how many challenges such an undertaking posed.

In a similar vein, Forum member Maryjoan Ladden from the Robert Wood Johnson Foundation acknowledged the long history of IPE, of which Ladden has been an active proponent since the 1970s. Educators have been trying for a long time to institute IPE and although momentum is growing, the many challenges have made it difficult. However, she said that she believes that the United States has a unique current opportunity to address neglected issues with the Affordable Care Act, the HRSA coordinated effort to develop a national clearinghouse, and the National Coordinating Center for Interprofessional Education and Collaborative Practice, which a group of funders has committed to supporting. It is also a good time, she said, to learn from the global conversations and the global partners in the Institute of Medicine Forum and to learn from the early adopters of IPE and collaborative care models. In the end, Ladden said she would like to learn what additional evidence chief executive officers of health systems and other key stakeholders need to be convinced of the value of collaborative care and of IPE and also what evidence early adopters of IPE need to provide to others to convince them to move forward?

Some of that evidence will likely come from the National Center for Interprofessional Practice and Education, initiated under Barbara Brandt. Although it was very early in the center's development, Brandt presented a description of the center at the workshop. She spoke about the plans for the center and how the idea for it grew out of the concern over a growing gap between the changing U.S. health system and health professions education. The center will focus on training in team-based care that improves health and community outcomes, she said. The particular outcomes they are interested in are grounded in the Institute for Healthcare Improvement's triple aim of improving the patient experience of care, improving the health of populations, and reducing the per capita cost of health care. The center will also be focusing on research and evidence to confirm the value added by its interventions. Box 7-1 offers a more detailed description of the center as described in Brandt's presentation.

Workshop II

As the final speaker of the second workshop, Martha Gaines said she would like to provide new ways of looking at old problems. Gaines is not a health professional. Rather, she is a lawyer by training, a former public defender, and a law professor for the past 25 years on the faculty at the University of Wisconsin Law School. Half of the years at the law school were spent with a prison program training students to work with prison inmates, and the other half were spent providing interprofessional education.

Nineteen years ago, she had a harrowing experience when she was diagnosed with metastatic ovarian cancer and told to go home and think about the quality, not the quantity, of her remaining days. At the time, her two children were ages 3 years and 6 months. After surviving the cancer, Gaines got together with a nurse, a physician, and two other colleagues and founded the Center for Patient Partnerships, an interdisciplinary center of the schools of law, medicine, nursing, and pharmacy at the University of Wisconsin. Gaines has been its director since its founding. The center advocates for people with life-threatening and serious chronic illnesses and educates graduates and health professionals about health advocacy. This was the context within which Gaines provided her reflective comments. She started by saying, "If the 20th century was about thinking the world apart because we have such amazing machines with which to make everything smaller and more microscopic, then I think the 21st century must be about thinking it back together again." Gaines said that it seems to her that this is the essence of IPE. It is "thinking the world back together again" so that the people who are meant to be served, namely patients and communities, can be something other than "the medication problem" that speaker Dennis Helling described.

Gaines listed some questions that came to her during the workshop. These included

- How does one approach working together when there is a lack of understanding about how the others work, what skills and knowledge they have, and what language they speak?
- What is IPE?
- How might it be known if IPE is delivering higher-quality and better care?
- Are there other models than IPE that could accomplish the same goals as well or better?
- Is there an ideal number of professions for IPE?
- Are there any irreplaceable professions within IPE?
- What is the minimum number of courses or programs needed to launch IPE?
- What are the roles for academics and practitioners in design and implementation?
- How is success defined?
- What is the value added from work in IPE?
- How has time for reflection been preserved?
- How has progress with other professionals been made?
- Who else needs to be part of the dialogue?
- What do university leaders think of health sciences education?
- Where are broader sources of support and resources?

In reflecting upon the last question, Gaines wondered how educators could connect with other similar movements to IPE to initiate new innovations. Thinking in this way could open a range of new possibilities for funding and collaborations.

Gaines also listed a number of important points that had particular resonance for her, as follows.

Take the Time to Be Intentional

When initiating IPE, take the time to form a mission and a vision, then share that mission and vision across interdisciplinary collaborations.

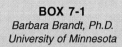

BOX 7-1
Barbara Brandt, Ph.D.
University of Minnesota

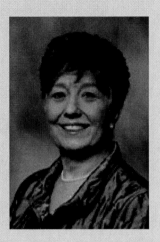

Barbara Brandt of the National Center for Interprofessional Practice and Education started her talk by acknowledging Hugh Barr, who she said was instrumental in transforming her thinking about IPE. In June 2008, Barr gave a presentation about IPE in Stockholm at the All Together Better Health conference in which he spoke about IPE in a way that differed from the usual thinking at the time. It was this transformed thinking, Brandt said, that serves as the underpinning for the National Center. Brandt explained that most people who worked in IPE were focused on teamwork and the patient safety agenda. It was Barr, she said, who pushed people to consider how interprofessional education could have a major impact on workforce development. And by combining health systems transformation with health professions transformation, interprofessional education could have an impact on both health and learning outcomes.

Another thing that happened in 2008 was that the state of Minnesota passed health care reform and was very aggressively implementing it. This was particularly significant to Brandt at the University of Minnesota. She noted that Minnesota has 197 certified health care or patient-centered medical homes, accountable care organizations, and other similar institutions. What that is demonstrating is that a gap is developing between health systems, which are undergoing a transformation, and health professions education in its current state. This was a message from Paul Grundy (the Global Director of IBM Healthcare Transformation) to the workshop participants that Brandt said she used as a focus of the National Center—the need for a more functional "nexus" between health systems and health professions education. The new nexus coming to team-based care, she said, focuses ultimately on improved health and community outcomes. The funded Health Resources and Services Administration (HRSA) proposal concentrated on the Institute for Healthcare Improvement's "triple aim," which consists of improving the patient experience of care, improving the health of populations, and reducing the per capita cost of health care.

Brandt then clarified that HRSA set the baseline rules for the National Center. These rules included having focuses on leadership, scholarship, evidence, coordination, and national visibility in order to advance interprofessional education and practice as a viable and efficient health care delivery model. It is a cooperative agreement, so she and her colleagues at the university are planning the center jointly with HRSA. HRSA is assisting Brandt by connecting the National Center with federal agencies that are working on health care reform, particularly the Center for Medicare and Medicaid Innovations, which has 104 projects being carried out throughout the United States. Another part of the work of the center involved HRSA's mandate: to transform a siloed U.S. health care system and to create new health care organizations; to facilitate the preparation of a workforce that is fully prepared through structured training and exposure; and to operate as a neutral and unbiased convener among stakeholders in education, practice, and public policy.

Because the primary funder for the center is HRSA, the center will focus on rural and underserved populations. As Minnesota's director of the statewide network of area health education centers, Brandt has a consortium of practice partners that she characterized as being an important underpinning of the proposal. Another group that had a prominent part in her proposal was Minnesota's Interprofessional Education and Collaborative Practice network, in which IPE is being implemented through the use of practice sites and the process of evaluating outcomes has begun. Evaluation was another key element in the proposal submitted to HRSA. The University of Minnesota has a fairly long history of evaluation through its Minnesota Evaluation Studies Institute. Brandt said that roughly 15 years ago the institute's evaluators developed essential competencies for program evaluators that have been translated worldwide. These evaluation experts are now looking at the center's vision to determine how their evaluation methods can be applied to interprofessional education and collaborative practice. Having reliable evaluation methods will be important as the center hopes to be a national innovation incubator for conducting research. This is extremely important to Brandt, who expressed her desire to get the metrics right.

Brandt then described the methodology framework used in the proposal. There are significant, uncoordinated activities going on in interprofessional education and collaborative practice. In an attempt to improve coordination, the center will be a central repository for relevant information that can be used in part to develop standards, definitions, measures, and protocols. Brandt also hopes to use informatics to connect patient electronic records with education and practice modalities to possibly evaluate the impact of IPE and interprofessional practice (IPP) on patient outcomes.

In her closing, Brandt described where she would like the center to be in 5 years. She envisions the center being connected with the world's best thinkers about IPE and IPP, who are fully engaged in the National Center's priority projects and who receive recognition for their work publicly across and within the professions. She wants public and private funders and partners to receive the highest return on investment possible. This includes making use of the latest technology and drawing conclusions from data that were collected and evaluated using rigorous evaluative processes. And finally, Brandt wants to see that the center makes significant contributions to improving health outcomes and to advancing the "triple aim."

Few Substitutes for Trusted Committed Leadership

There is little substitute for passion and commitment by a person or people with vision. And when inspiration does not come from leadership, the people who have the passion and commitment will have to "manage up" to explain and demonstrate the value of IPE to their leadership. This can be done by sharing stories, gathering evidence, and building a network with other champions.

Adverse Conditions Create Opportunities for Change

Gaines pointed to the example from Ghent University's medical school described earlier, when a bad evaluation was the needed spark for movement from a fragmented, discipline-based curriculum to what is now an integrated patient- and problem-based curriculum.

Learn More About Culture Change

Much has been written about disciplinary and cross-disciplinary culture (Dee Fink, 2003; Zajonc, 2008; Palmer, 2010), Gaines said. Learning more about culture change through the literature and from personal experiences will help students, educators, and professionals become more astute agents for positive cultural changes.

Lack of IPE Measurements

There is a lack of evidence, data, and proof of the value of IPE. Gaines emphasized that the value proposition—or the assessment of value—can be strengthened by including that which is not traditionally considered in the evaluation of the bottom-line cost–benefit equation. Such things might include workforce morale, patient satisfaction, a life well-lived, inspiration, or excitement about doing a job. Those are all things that could be inserted into the evaluation equation to get a better sense of the value of IPE and collaborative work.

It Is Hard to Learn Publicly

Gaines gave one description of teaching as "to learn publicly." This is difficult to do and horribly embarrassing. Fear of others knowing that the expert is not the expert in all things can be a source of apprehension for those who are engaging in new processes, such as IPE. By establishing learning communities that bring together different professions across the continuum of education to practice to better understand IPE, could be an important leveler of hierarchies and a way of breaking free from conventional stereotypes.

Create Value for the Learning Sites

Gaines commented that speaker Mark Earnest had talked about "value-added learners." If learning sites viewed students as adding value to their work, this would likely lead to more sustainable relationships between education and practice. It would also be better for students who gain from the experiential learning.

Plagiarize with Pride

Although educators do not like using the word "plagiarize" in academia, Gaines said, it is generally accepted that in IPE educators should imitate the work of others rather than reinvent that which has already been tested. As an example, Gaines pointed to speaker Dawn Forman and others who talked about drawing on previous IPE efforts to come up with formulas that work at their own universities.

Listen to Nontraditional Sources of Ideas and Innovation

Gaines noted the creative interprofessional ideas that had been presented at the workshop but had not come from faculty. In particular, she cited speaker Lloyd Michener, who commented that solutions are often driven by students. She also described the potentially underutilized value of others, such as front office staff and janitorial hospital workers. These nonprofessionals may be in a better position to connect with people and patients in a unique way, and this could be a tremendous resource for collaborative work.

Create and Protect Space to Reflect

Gaines noted that some of the student presenters had commented that social interactions for establishing personal relationships are just as important for learning about other professions and cultures as the physical space and time to interact with the other health professions.

IPE Is Best When It Is Memorable

Gaines noted students' comments about the value of memorable IPE that is interactive both professionally and personally and in which education and practice are linked.

Harmonize Academic Calendars

Harmonizing academic calendars could be one way to better ensure representations of more professions in IPE. At least one student, Gaines noted, had identified the absence of other health professional learners as an impediment to her IPE.

IPE Is a High-Touch Learning Environment

Several participants spoke of the need to engage educators beyond the faculty because IPE a high-touch learning environment. For example, Gaines said, speaker Rose Nabirye talked about how problems arise when the number of students is too high and not everyone gets access in a way that he or she believes is meaningful.

Gaines closed her remarks by posing four questions to the workshop participants. The first involved engaging patients in designing, planning, evaluating, and promoting IPE. If patients think it is important to be involved with educating the next generation of health professionals—and assuming professionals do as well—then why is it still so rare for patients to be engaged across the continuum not just in IPE, but across education and across service delivery as well? Her second question was, "How should educators handle students who are not so enthusiastic about IPE?" Gaines suggested that maybe educators will have to make IPE a mandatory requirement for graduation. But that assumes the interprofessional experience is intentionally grounded in the context of students' lives, because it is when the experience is based in real-life practice that value is added to students' education.

The third question Gaines posed was "What holds educators and health professionals back from letting go of traditional models of care?" This may, she suggested, be tied to feelings of identity and a fear of losing the history and stories linked to professional heroes and heroines that make each profession unique. Her fourth and final question was "Should a social mission be a mandatory part of health professions education?" Gaines thought that addressing social determinants of health would bring in additional disciplines such as social work and law, which would lead to a wider impact on various health outcomes but would increase the complexity of the team possibly presenting new challenges in management for both the student and the IPE coordinator.

Transformative Health Professional Education and IPE

In his reflective comments on the workshop, Forum and planning committee member Jan De Maesaneer from Ghent University in Belgium commented that social accountability will lead to transformative health professional education and changes resulting in greater equity. At one point during the workshop, De Maesaneer was asked to define "transformative health professional education." Although it is not easy, De Maesaneer said, he did attempt to come up a definition, and the result was as follows:

> Transformative health professional education is a process. It occurs when institutions for health professional education respond to the needs of the population through a series of socially accountable change actions aimed at three levels—the micro, the meso, and the macro. The micro level focuses on educational transformations to help prepare health care providers to practice more person- and people-centered care, combining appropriate knowledge and skills training in a process of self-directed caring, to what is reflective practice. The meso level involves interactions with health services, providers, and citizens in the community, including the establishment of community-based training complexes that emphasize those areas most in need—like deprived rural and urban environments. At the macro level, there would be active participation in processes of health policy development with special attention to human resources spending and contributions that make health systems worldwide increasingly based on relevance, equity, quality, cost effectiveness, system ability, person- and people-centeredness, and innovation.

De Maeseneer's definition of transformative health professional education had clear links to Paul Worley's closing comments. In those comments Worley said he thought that the workshop had provided an excellent reflection on interprofessional education and that participants had discovered not only that cultures can change and practical bottlenecks should be overcome, but that interprofessional education is needed and that it is possible to make it happen now. He said that he had also learned that for this to be accomplished, there will need to be a transformative process that involves patients and populations, the educational system, and the health system; excellent examples exist that were described in this workshop for all to learn from.

To find out more about the workshops discussed in this report, please visit the Global Forum on Innovation in Health Professional Education website at www.iom.edu/IHPEGlobalForum.

REFERENCES

Dee Fink, L. 2003. *Creating significant learning experiences.* Hoboken, NJ: Jossey-Bass.

Palmer, P. 2010. *The violence of our knowledge: Toward a spirituality of higher education.* http://www.21learn.org (accessed March 12, 2013).

WHO (World Health Organization). 1978. *Declaration of Alma-Ata.* Geneva: WHO.

WHO. 1981. *Global strategy for health for all by the year 2000.* Geneva: WHO.

Zajonc, A. 2008. *Meditation as contemplative inquiry: When knowing becomes love.* Aurora, CO: Lindisfarne Press.

A

Workshop Agendas

A Workshop Series of the Institute of Medicine
Global Forum on Innovation in Health Professional Education
(IHPE Global Forum)

**Workshop I: Interprofessional Education for Collaboration:
Learning How to Improve Health from Interprofessional
Models Across the Continuum of Education to Practice**

August 29–30, 2012

The Keck Center of The National Academies
500 Fifth Street, NW
Washington, DC 20001
Room 100

Workshop Objectives:

- To engage in forward-looking dialogue around the importance of aligning health professional education with the needs of clinical practice, consumers, and the health care delivery system;
- To explore the opportunity for shared decision making, distributed leadership, and team-based care, amongst other interprofessional education (IPE) and practice innovations, to fundamentally change health professions curriculums, pedagogy, culture, human resources, and assessment and evaluation metrics; and
- To discuss how innovations in IPE will impact patient and population health as identified through the "triple aim" of better health, higher quality, and lower cost.

DAY 1: AUGUST 29, 2012

9:00 a.m.   **Welcome and Introductions**
Scott Reeves, *Workshop Planning Committee Co-Chair*
Lucinda Maine, *Workshop Planning Committee Co-Chair*

9:15 a.m.   **Why Focus on IPE as a Key Health Professions Education Innovation?**
Objective: To frame the importance of better alignment between health professions education and the needs for better health, better care, and lower costs.
George Thibault, Josiah Macy Jr. Foundation
Q & A

10:00 a.m.   **Panel Discussion: Making the Case for the Integration of Practice Redesign and Education Reform**
Objectives: To offer a variety of perspectives about how health professions education for shared decision making, distributed leadership, and team-based care can improve health delivery systems' positive impact on individual and population health outcomes; and to examine to what extent health professional education is currently meeting these kinds of practice needs.
Moderator: Matt Wynia, Institute for Ethics, American Medical Association
Panelists:
- Interprofessional practice: Craig Jones, Vermont Blueprint for Health
- Education reform: Barbara Brandt, University of Minnesota Academic Health Center
- Student: Sandeep Kishore, Young Professionals Chronic Disease Working Group
Respondents:
- Patient perspective: Rosemary Gibson, Author, *Wall of Silence, Archives of Internal Medicine*
- Employer perspective: Paul Grundy, IBM Healthcare Transformation
Q & A

12:00 p.m.   **LUNCH**

1:00 p.m. **White Paper Presentation**
Objective: To lay the foundation for the small-group discussions around actualizing educational reform relevant to practice in the five areas for innovation—curriculum, pedagogy, metrics, culture, and resources—using elements of the triple aim as the outcome focus.
Lucinda Maine, *Co-Chair*
Q & A

2:00 p.m. **Small-Group Breakout Sessions Instructions**
Lucinda Maine, *Co-Chair*

Using an appreciative inquiry approach, address the following questions:
- What are the strengths and opportunities in using IPE to improve practice through better health, better care, better access, or lower costs?
- Using curricular redesign, pedagogical innovation, culture, metrics, and human resources, how do we drive IPE competencies (and beyond?) toward the outcomes captured in the triple aims (better health, higher quality, lower cost)?

Additional guidance:
- Could discuss these IPE questions focusing on any educational stage along the learning continuum from undergraduate/prelicensure to continuing education.
- Can consider non-professionals insofar as professionals learn to interact with non-professionals as part of the team as well as other professionals.
- Provide specific examples of places where IPE educational innovations in the five areas are designed to impact health, care, access, or costs.

2:30 p.m. **Break into Small Groups**
Objectives: To explore opportunities for improving health, care, access, or lower costs through the use of IPE in the areas of curricular innovations, pedagogic innovations, cultural elements, human resources for health, and metrics that positively impact the triple aim; to identify exemplars and best practices that are already applying such innovations; and to identify

gaps where IPE could be used to achieve better health, care, or access or lower costs, but where it is not yet being applied, and brainstorm strategies for promoting implementation in these areas.

1. Better health
   - Group leader: Pamela Jeffries, Johns Hopkins University School of Nursing
     Assistance by Harrison Spencer, Workshop Planning Committee member
2. Better care (higher quality using teamwork and shared decision making)
   - Group leader: Lorna Lynn, American Board of Internal Medicine
     Assistance by Brenda Zierler, Workshop Planning Committee member
3. Enhanced access (enhanced access to education of patients/populations as learners and educators of team-based, collaborative care)
   - Group leader: Sally Okun, PatientsLikeMe
     Assistance by Mattie Schmitt, Workshop Planning Committee member
4. Lower cost
   - Group leader: Thomas Feeley, MD Anderson Cancer Center
     Assistance by George Thibault, Workshop Planning Committee member

4:00 p.m.   **BREAK (reconvene in large group)**

4:30 p.m.   **Debriefing of Small-Group Session**
Moderator: Scott Reeves, *Co-Chair*

4:45 p.m.   **Canadian Interprofessional Health Leadership Collaborative**
Objective: To provide a case study from the Global Forum's Canadian Interprofessional Health Leadership Collaborative describing how IPE is being linked to practice.
Linking Health Professions Education to Practice: Canadian Successes and Lessons Learned
- Sarita Verma, Co-Lead, Canadian Interprofessional Health Leadership Collaborative

> • Maria Tassone, Co-Lead, Canadian
> Interprofessional Health Leadership Collaborative
> Q & A

5:30 p.m.   **ADJOURN**

DAY 2: AUGUST 30, 2012

8:00 a.m.   **Breakfast and Report by Three Regional Collaboratives
in India, Uganda, and South Africa**
Moderator: Patrick Kelley, Director of Board on Global
Health
• Sanjay Zodpey, India Collaborative
• Nelson Sewankambo, Uganda Collaborative
• Marietjie de Villiers, South Africa Collaborative
Q & A panel discussion

9:00 a.m.   **Recap of Day 1**
Scott Reeves, *Co-Chair*

9:15 a.m.   **Small-Group Report Back**
Moderator: Patricia Hinton Walker, Uniformed Services
University of the Health Sciences
• Pamela Jeffries, Johns Hopkins University School of
Nursing
• Lorna Lynn, American Board of Internal Medicine
• Sally Okun, PatientsLikeMe
• Thomas Feeley, MD Anderson Cancer Center
Q & A panel discussion with small-group leaders

10:00 a.m.   **BREAK**

10:15 a.m.   **Reflection Panel**
*Objectives: To reflect on the Day 1 discussions in an
effort to identify principles of effective IPE and gaps
that inhibit effective IPE, and to provide insight from
different perspectives on how to better link health
professional education with practice moving forward,
including what currently is working to further this goal
and what the priority areas for investment might be.*

Moderator: Brenda Zierler, University of Washington
- Patient perspective: Brigid Vaughan
- Employer of health workers: Marilyn Chow, Kaiser Permanente
- Philanthropy: Gillian Barclay, Aetna Foundation
- Population health: John Finnegan, University of Minnesota

Q & A panel discussion

11:45 a.m.   **Closing Address**
Social accountability in medical education: An Australian rural and remote perspective
Paul Worley, Dean of the School of Medicine at Flinders University, Australia

12:15 p.m.   **Summative Comments and the Way Forward**
Moderator: Scott Reeves, *Co-Chair*
- Maryjoan Ladden, Robert Wood Johnson Foundation, Forum member
- Jan De Maeseneer, Workshop II planning committee member
- Mattie Schmitt, Workshop I and II planning committee member

Open forum discussion

1:00 p.m.   **LUNCH/ADJOURN**

Workshop II: Interprofessional Education for Collaboration:
Learning How to Improve Health from Interprofessional
Models Across the Continuum of Education to Practice

November 29–30, 2012

The Keck Center of The National Academies
500 Fifth Street, NW
Washington, DC 20001
Room 100

Workshop Objectives:

- To derive principles and lessons learned from sustained and exemplar IPE models across the continuum of education;
- To identify and examine academic/practice partnerships that demonstrate purposeful modeling to advance team-based education and collaborative practice; and
- To learn from IPE exemplars across the education/practice continuum that link to better health, higher quality, and improved value for individuals and populations.

DAY 1: NOVEMBER 29, 2012

8:00 a.m.   **Breakfast**

8:30 a.m.   **Welcome and Introductions**
              Introduction by Afaf Meleis, *IHPE Global Forum Co-Chair*
              - Lucinda Maine, *Workshop II Co-Chair*
              - Scott Reeves, *Workshop II Co-Chair*

8:40 a.m.   **Opening Address**
              Introduction by Jordan Cohen, *IHPE Global Forum Co-Chair*
              - Samuel Thier, Professor Emeritus, Health Care Policy and Medicine, Harvard Medical School

9:10 a.m.   **New National Coordinating Center (NCC) for IPE and IPP-University of Minnesota**
              - Barbara Brandt, NCC Director

9:35 a.m.   **IPE as an Educational Innovation: Overview of Principles and Lessons Learned**
Objectives: To derive principles and lessons learned about initiation and sustainability of IPE and how IPE success is measured.
Moderator: Hugh Barr, President of the U.K. Centre for the Advancement of Interprofessional Education (CAIPE)
- University of Colorado
  o Mark Earnest, Director, Interprofessional Education
- Curtin University, Perth, Australia
  o Dawn Forman, Professor of Interprofessional Education and Clinical Director (via video conference)
- Linköping University, Sweden
  o Margaretha Wilhelmsson, Vice Director of Study, Faculty of Health Science

10:45 a.m.   **BREAK**

11:15 a.m.   **IPE as an Educational Innovation: Principles and Lessons Learned for Linking IPE to Educational and Practice Outcomes**
Objectives: To learn from IPE exemplars that strive to link to better health, higher quality, and improved value for individuals and populations and how IPE success is measured.
Moderator: John Tegzes, Director of IPE, Western University of Health Sciences
- Kaiser Permanente Colorado Region, Department of Pharmacy
  o Dennis Helling, Executive Director, Pharmacy Operations & Therapeutics
- University of Missouri
  o Carla Dyer, Faculty Lead on IPE
- Ghent University, Belgium
  o Jan De Maeseneer, Head, Department of Family Medicine and Primary Health Care
- Thomas Jefferson University
  o Elizabeth Speakman, Co-Director, Jefferson Interprofessional Education Center

12:30 p.m.   **LUNCH**

1:15 p.m.   **Student Session: Learning from the Learners**
               Objective: To gain a better understanding of how
               students view IPE and what aspects of IPE/IPP do or do
               not resonate with them as learners.
               What is it like to go through an IPE curriculum?
               What is your perspective on IPE—what resonates and
               what does not?
               Moderator: Mohammed Ali, Assistant Professor at
               Emory's Hubert Department of Global Health and
               member of the Young Professionals Chronic Disease
               Network (YP-CDN)
                 • Student 1: Erin Abu-Rish, Multidisciplinary
                   Predoctoral Clinical Research Training Program
                   Trainee, University of Washington School of
                   Nursing
                 • Student 2: Edward Thomas Lewis, Resident
                   Physician, Department of Psychiatry, Medical
                   University of South Carolina
                 • Student 3: Jenny Wong, College of Pharmacy,
                   University of Minnesota
                 • Student 4: Angella Namwase, 2nd Year Bachelor
                   of Nursing Student, Makerere University (via video
                   conference)
               Q & A panel discussion

2:15 p.m.   **Move to Small-Group Room Assignment**

2:25 p.m.   **Small-Group Breakouts**
               Objective: To further examine dimensions of successful
               relationships between education and practice across the
               interprofessional education continuum.
               Group 1: What are the local, institutional, and national
               factors driving the initiation of collaborative partnerships
               between interprofessional education and practice?
               Leader: Warren Newton, Vice Dean of Education for
               University of North Carolina School of Medicine, Family
               Medicine

Group 2: What makes collaboration between education and practice for IPE successful and sustainable (support your conclusions with exemplars across the continuum of education from classroom to practice)?

Leader: Donna Meyer, President, National Organization for Associate Degree Nursing

Group 3: How should the outcomes of interprofessional education be measured/assessed assuming the ultimate goal is better health, higher quality, and improved value for individual patients and populations?
Leader: Eric Holmboe, Chief Medical Officer and Senior Vice President, American Board of Internal Medicine

Group 4: How does one get buy-in from leadership when initiating or sustaining IPE/IPP (including linking education and practice from either perspective)?
Leader: Hugh Barr, President of the U.K. Centre for the Advancement of Interprofessional Education (CAIPE)

4:00 p.m.   **Return to Main Room**

4:15 p.m.   Debriefing with entire group (discuss general issues that arose during the small-group sessions)
Moderator: Lucinda Maine, *Workshop II Co-Chair*

4:40 p.m.   Canadian Collaborative
   • Collaborative Representatives: Sarita Verma and Maria Tassone, Co-Leads

5:00 p.m.   **ADJOURN**

DAY 2: NOVEMBER 30, 2012

8:00 a.m.   **Breakfast and Report by Two Country Collaboratives**
Moderator: Patrick Kelley, IOM Director, Board on Global Health
   • Rose Nabirye, Makerere University, Uganda
   • Stefanus Snyman, Stellenbosch University, South Africa

9:00 a.m.   **Leaders of the Small Groups Report Back**
               Moderator: Geraldine Polly Bednash, American
               Association of Colleges of Nursing
                   • Q & A panel discussion with small-group leaders

9:30 a.m.   **BREAK**

9:50 a.m.   **Practice Session: Integrating Students into
               Interprofessional Practice**
               *Objective: To identify opportunities and challenges for
               student placements and projects in team-based models.*
               How might academia and practice work together to create
               viable models for placing students across the educational
               continuum in high-functioning, interprofessional teams?
               Moderator: Malcolm Cox, Chief Academic Affiliations
               Officer, U.S. Department of Veterans Affairs
                   • David Collier, Director, Pediatric Healthy Weight
                     Research and Treatment Center, Department
                     of Pediatrics, Brody School of Medicine at East
                     Carolina University
                   • Steven Chen, Associate Professor of Clinical
                     Pharmacy serving in University of Southern
                     California (USC) safety-net clinics

10:50 a.m.   **"STRETCH YOUR LEGS" BREAK**

11:00 a.m.   **Learning from "Exemplar" Academic/Practice
               Partnerships**
               *Objective: To identify and examine academic/practice
               partnerships that demonstrate purposeful modeling to
               advance team-based education and collaborative practice.*
               Moderator: Lisa Lehmann, Director, Center for Bioethics,
               Brigham & Women's Hospital, Associate Professor of
               Medicine and Medical Ethics, Harvard Medical School
                   • Kathryn Rugen, Nurse Consultant, Veterans Affairs
                     Centers of Excellence in Primary Care Education
                   • Valentina Brashers, Professor of Nursing and
                     Attending Physician in Internal Medicine,
                     University of Virginia

12:00 p.m.   **Keynote**
                Introduction by Harrison Spencer, Association of Schools
                and Programs of Public Health
                  • James Lloyd Michener, Professor and Chair of the
                    Department of Community and Family Medicine,
                    Duke University Medical Center

12:30 p.m.   **Summary and Assessment**
                  • Martha Gaines, Associate Dean for Academic
                    Affairs and Experiential Learning; Director of
                    Center for Patient Partnership, University of
                    Wisconsin

1:00 p.m.   **LUNCH/ADJOURN**

B

Speaker Biographies

Erin Abu-Rish, M.A., is a nurse with a background in community health, public and social policy, and interprofessional education (IPE). She is currently a fourth-year Ph.D. student at the University of Washington (UW) School of Nursing, where she is a National Institutes of Health–funded trainee in the Multidisciplinary Predoctoral Clinical Research Training Program of UW's Institute of Translational Health Sciences. For her dissertation research, Ms. Abu-Rish is collaborating with the Public Health Activities and Services Tracking Study to focus on exploring relationships among the recent economic downturn, public health budget cuts at the local health department level, and individual-level maternal and child health outcomes and disparities. Since 2009 she has worked as a graduate research assistant on IPE training grants. She also helped to establish the UW Health Science Students Institute for Healthcare Improvement Open School Chapter.

Mohammed Ali, M.B.Ch.B., M.Sc., M.B.A., is an assistant professor of global health at Emory University and IPA consultant for the Division of Diabetes Translation at the U.S. Centers for Disease Control and Prevention (CDC). He is a co-investigator for three studies in India: a large surveillance study, a case-control study investigating early onset diabetes, and a translation trial of comprehensive care for people with diabetes. He is a working group member for a quality of life and costs of care assessment (the ACCORD study). He also co-leads the expert group on diabetes complications for the Global Burden of Disease Study. At the CDC, Dr. Ali helps manage a collaborative network of investigators (the NEXT-D Study) that evaluates the effects of different policy changes on diabetes prevention and control and that provides scientific advice for the National Diabetes Prevention Program. He also works actively with Emory's Global Health Institute as a senior fellow and directs the institute's signature Global Health Case Competition.

Gillian Barclay, D.D.S., Dr.P.H., is vice president of programs of the Aetna Foundation. In her role she leads the development, execution, and evaluation of the foundation's national grant programs and cultivates new projects within its three focus areas: reducing obesity, improving health care equity, and promoting integrated health care. As part of her responsibilities, she also is a frequent spokesperson for the foundation, presenting its work and the accomplishments of grantees to internal and external constituents. Prior to joining the Aetna Foundation, Dr. Barclay was an advisor for the regional office of the World Health Organization in the Office of Caribbean Program Coordination. In that position she managed a portfolio of health initiatives in the region that focused special attention on the impact of gender, human rights, integrated health systems, and essential public health functions on access to quality health care. Previously she was the evaluation manager of health programs for the W.K. Kellogg Foundation, responsible for assessing the foundation's health initiatives in the areas of reducing health disparities, community- and school-based health care, and oral health, among others.

Hugh Barr, M.Phil., Ph.D., is president of the U.K. Centre for the Advancement of Interprofessional Education and emeritus editor of the *Journal of Interprofessional Care*. He was awarded his Ph.D. by the University of Greenwich based on his interprofessional publications and honorary doctorates by East Anglia and Southampton universities and honorary fellowship from the University of Westminster for his role in promoting interprofessional education (IPE) nationally and internationally. His publications in that field include surveys, practice guidelines, and systematic reviews. He served on the World Health Organization study group on IPE and collaborative practice. His background is in probation, prison aftercare, criminology, and social work education.

Geraldine "Polly" Bednash, Ph.D., R.N., FAAN, was appointed executive director of the American Association of Colleges of Nursing (AACN) in 1989. Prior to serving as executive director and chief executive officer, Dr. Bednash headed the association's legislative and regulatory advocacy programs as director of government affairs. In that post from 1986 to 1989, she directed AACN's efforts to secure strong federal support for nursing education and research, coordinated new initiatives with federal agencies and with major foundations, and coauthored AACN's landmark study of the financial costs to students and to clinical agencies of baccalaureate and graduate nursing education. Dr. Bednash currently serves as chair of the Nursing Alliance for Quality Care, as a member of the Sullivan Alliance to Transform the Health Professions, and as a member of the Quality Alliance Steering Committee. Additionally, she has been appointed to the Secretary's Academic Affiliations Council of the Department of Veterans Affairs.

Barbara F. Brandt, Ph.D., has served as the associate vice president for education and as a professor of pharmaceutical care and health systems at the University of Minnesota Academic Health Center since 2000. She has served as the principal investigator and director of the Minnesota Area Health Education Center statewide network, an interprofessional workforce development program for rural and urban underserved in Minnesota. Dr. Brandt is responsible for implementing the University of Minnesota Academic Health Center 1Health initiative in interprofessional education in allied health, dentistry, medicine, nursing, pharmacy, public health, and veterinary medicine.

Valentina Brashers, M.D., is professor of nursing, Woodard Clinical Scholar, and attending physician in internal medicine at the University of Virginia (UVA). After completing her residency in internal medicine and a fellowship in pulmonary disease, she practiced in a rural general medical clinic and in the UVA emergency room. She is a founding member of the UVA School of Medicine Academy of Distinguished Educators and is the first physician to be elected as an honorary member of the UVA Nursing Alumni Association. She is the first professor to win the UVA All University Outstanding Teaching Award twice, and she has received the Excellence in Teaching Award from both the UVA School of Nursing and the UVA School of Medicine. Dr. Brashers is the founder and co-chair of the UVA Interprofessional Education Initiative, which provides leadership and oversight to more than 25 interprofessional education experiences for students and faculty at all levels of training.

Steven W. Chen, Pharm.D., is an associate professor at the University of Southern California (USC) School of Pharmacy and a licensed pharmacist. Dr. Chen holds the Hygeia Centennial Chair in Clinical Pharmacy at USC for his work and leadership in improving medication use and safety in the community through clinical pharmacy services in safety net clinics. In addition, he has received several national awards for his work to improve medication use and safety in uninsured, vulnerable populations receiving care in federally qualified health centers and safety net clinics in the Los Angeles community as well as at Cedars-Sinai Medical Center.

Marilyn Chow, R.N., D.N.Sc., is the vice president of national patient care services at Kaiser Permanente, where she works with nursing leaders and senior executives across all regions and collaborates with internal and external partners to enable the delivery of the highest quality and safest patient-centered care. Her career has focused on promoting the role of nurses in primary care, advanced practice, and hospital-based care. Dr. Chow is committed to incorporating innovation and technology to reduce waste and improve workflows within the health care industry. She was the driving force in conceptualizing and creating the Garfield Innovation Center, Kaiser Permanente's living laboratory, where ideas are tested and solutions are developed in a hands-on, simulated clinical environment.

David N. Collier, M.D., Ph.D., is an associate professor of pediatrics and adjunct associate professor of family medicine and kinesiology at the Brody School of Medicine at East Carolina University (ECU). He is also director of ECU's Pediatric Healthy Weight Research and Treatment Center, an associate director for the East Carolina Diabetes and Obesity Institute, and vice chair for research for the Department of Pediatrics. His clinical and research interests are focused on understanding the causes and consequences of childhood obesity.

Malcolm Cox, M.D., is the chief academic affiliations officer for the Veterans Administration (VA), where he oversees the largest health professions education program in the United States. Previously he was chief of medicine at the Philadelphia VA Medical Center, associate dean for clinical education at the University of Pennsylvania, and dean for medical education at Harvard Medical School. During the past 5 years, Dr. Cox has led a major expansion of the VA's medical, nursing, and associated health training programs and an intensive reevaluation of the VA's educational infrastructure and affiliation relationships. At the same time he has repositioned the Office of Academic Affiliations as a major voice in health professions workforce reform and educational innovation. Dr. Cox currently serves on the Strategic Directions Committee of the National Leadership Council of the Veterans Health Administration, the National Advisory Committee of the Robert Wood Johnson Clinical Scholars Program, the National Board of Medical Examiners, and the Accreditation Council for Graduate Medical Education.

Jan De Maeseneer, M.D., Ph.D., has been working as a family physician in the community health center Botermarkt in Ledeberg, a deprived area in the city of Ghent, Belgium. Since 2008 he has served as vice dean for strategic planning on the Faculty of Medicine and Health Sciences. He is board member of the Interuniversity Flemish Consortium for vocational training of family medicine, and he chairs the working party for family medicine of the Belgian High Council for medical specialists and family physicians. Professor De Maeseneer chairs the Educational Committee (since 1997) and directs a fundamental reform of the undergraduate curriculum (from a discipline-based to an integrated patient-based approach). In 2004 Professor De Maeseneer received the WONCA-Award for Excellence in Health Care: The Five-Star Doctor at the 17th World Conference of Family Doctors in Orlando, Florida. In 2008 he received a Doctor Honoris Causa degree at the Universidad Mayor de San Simon in Cochabamba, Bolivia. In 2010 he received the prize De Schaepdrijver-Caenepeel for developmental work from the Royal Flemish Academy of Medicine.

Marietjie de Villiers, Ph.D., M.B.Ch.B., M.Fam.Med., is deputy dean of education at the Faculty of Health Sciences (FHS) of Stellenbosch University in South Africa, where she is also a professor in family medicine and primary care. She is currently responsible for all curriculum development, educational innovation, program implementation, and quality assurance on undergraduate, postgraduate, and continuing education levels at the FHS. Professor de Villiers is chairperson of the Stellenbosch University Rural Medical Education Partnership Advisory Committee and is actively involved in the implementation and evaluation of the Medical Education Partnership Initiative.

Carla Dyer, M.D., associate clinical professor of internal medicine and child health, is a Med-Peds hospitalist physician and clerkship director for the department of internal medicine at the University of Missouri. She directs the Introduction to Patient Care courses for the University of Missouri School of Medicine students. She chairs the Interprofessional Curriculum in Quality and Safety steering committee and led the development of an interprofessional simulation focused on patient safety. She collaborates with School of Nursing and School of Pharmacy faculty to develop and integrate interprofessional learning opportunities for health professional students. Her research interests include interprofessional education, patient safety, quality improvement education for health professional students, and simulation.

Mark Earnest, M.D., Ph.D., is a professor of medicine at the University of Colorado's Anschutz Medical Campus, where he teaches and practices internal medicine. Dr. Earnest is the director of interprofessional education at the University of Colorado Anschutz Medical Campus, where he oversees the REACH Program (Realizing Educational Advancement in Collaborative Health). REACH involves students from all the health profession programs on campus in a longitudinal curriculum designed to improve quality and safety of care through more effective interprofessional collaboration and teamwork. The program is funded by grants from the Josiah Macy Jr. Foundation and the Colorado Health Foundation. Dr. Earnest serves on the board of the American Interprofessional Health Collaborative and also founded and directs the LEADS track (Leadership Education Advocacy Development Scholarship)—a track within the school of medicine that develops leadership skills with an emphasis on service to the community and civic engagement.

Thomas W. Feeley, M.D., is the Helen Shafer Fly Distinguished Professor of Anesthesiology and head of the Division of Anesthesiology and Critical Care at the University of Texas MD Anderson Cancer Center. He has led MD Anderson's Institute for Cancer Care Excellence since its formation in 2008. The Institute for Cancer Care Excellence focuses on research to improve the value of cancer care delivery through programs that measure outcomes and costs of cancer care delivery. Dr. Feeley currently serves on the Institute of Medicine's Committee on Improving the Quality of Cancer Care: Addressing the Challenges of an Aging Population.

Dawn Forman, Ph.D., M.B.A., is currently professor of interprofessional education and clinical director at Curtin University, Perth, Australia. She uses her coaching skills as a leader and manager within the organization and with key stakeholders to facilitate change and new ways of working. Dr. Forman is internationally recognized in her field and widely published. In addition to her work at Curtin University. Dr. Forman is currently visiting professor at the University of Chichester (U.K.) and adjunct professor at Auckland University of Technology (New Zealand).

Martha (Meg) Gaines, J.D., L.L.M., is the associate dean for academic affairs and experiential learning at the University of Wisconsin Law School, where she has served as a clinical professor of law for 25 years. She is also founding director of the interdisciplinary Center for Patient Partnerships, which trains future professionals in medicine, nursing, law, health systems, industrial engineering, pharmacy, genetic counseling, and other disciplines who provide advocacy services to patients with life-threatening and serious chronic illnesses. Ms. Gaines teaches courses related to consumer issues in health care advocacy to graduate students pursuing various health professions and law. Following her graduation from law school, she served as a law clerk to the late Hon. Thomas Tang, 9th Circuit Court of Appeals and as a trial attorney for the Wisconsin State Public Defender.

Rosemary Gibson, M.Sc., is a national leader in health care quality and safety and a section editor of the *Archives of Internal Medicine*'s "Less is More" series. She is principal author of the new book *The Battle Over*

Health Care: What Obama's Health Care Reform Means for America's Future, a non-partisan analysis of the future state of health care and its impact on the economy. Ms. Gibson led national health care quality and safety initiatives at the Robert Wood Johnson Foundation for 16 years. She was the chief architect of the foundation's decade-long strategy to establish palliative care in the mainstream of the U.S. health care system. Ms. Gibson is the author of the critically acclaimed book *Wall of Silence*, which tells the human story behind the Institute of Medicine report *To Err Is Human*, and *The Treatment Trap*, a book on the overuse of medical care. She is a graduate of Georgetown University and has a master's degree from the London School of Economics.

Paul Grundy, M.D., M.P.H., FACOEM, FACPM, is one of only 38 IBM employees and the only physician selected into IBM's senior industry leadership forum, known as the IBM Industry Academy. Prior to joining IBM, Dr. Grundy worked as a senior diplomat in the U.S. Department of State supporting the intersection of health and diplomacy. He was also medical director for the International SOS, the world's largest medical assistance company, and for Adventist Health Systems, the second largest not-for-profit medical system in the world. Dr. Grundy is the president of the Patient-Centered Primary Care Collaborative and is an adjunct professor at the University of Utah's Department of Family and Preventive Medicine. He was made an honorary member of the American Academy of Family and has won three Department of State superior honor awards and four Department of State meritorious service awards.

Dennis K. Helling, Pharm.D., D.Sc., is executive director of pharmacy operations and therapeutics at Kaiser Permanente, Denver. His department employs more than 900 staff at its 37 pharmacies, emphasizing expanded roles for pharmacists and ambulatory clinical services. Dr. Helling's department is recognized nationally and internationally for innovative pharmacy services in managed care. He is a clinical professor at the University of Colorado School of Pharmacy and has been elected fellow of the American College of Clinical Pharmacology (ACCP) and the American Society of Health-System Pharmacists. Dr. Helling was a founding member and president of ACCP and president of the American Council for Pharmacy Education. During his 19 years in academia Dr. Helling was the associate dean for clinical affairs and professor and chair in the Department of Pharmacy Practice at the University of Houston and associate professor and head in the Division of Clinical/Hospital Pharmacy at the University of Iowa. Dr. Helling currently serves as vice president of the Denver Hospice board of directors and is immediate past president of the American Pharmacists Association Foundation. His practice emphasis and research have focused on documenting the impact pharmacists have on improving patient outcomes and the costs of health care.

Eric Holmboe, M.D., a board-certified internist, is chief medical officer and senior vice president of the American Board of Internal Medicine (ABIM) and the ABIM Foundation. He is also professor adjunct of medicine at Yale University and adjunct professor at the Uniformed Services University of the Health Sciences. Previously he was associate program director of the Yale Primary Care Internal Medicine Residency Program and director of Student Clinical Assessment at the Yale School of Medicine. Before joining Yale he was division chief of General Internal Medicine at the National Naval Medical Center. His research interests include interventions to improve quality of care and methods in the evaluation of clinical competence. Dr. Holmboe is a member of the National Board of Medical Examiners and Medbiquitous and is a consultant for the Drug Safety and Risk Management Subcommittee of the Pharmaceutical Science Advisory Committee for the U.S. Food and Drug Administration. He is a fellow of the American College of Physicians and an honorary fellow of the Royal College of Physicians in London.

Pamela R. Jeffries, Ph.D., R.N., A.N.E.F., FAAN, is the associate dean of academic affairs at Johns Hopkins School of Nursing. She has more than 25 years of teaching experience in the classroom, learning laboratory, and clinical setting with undergraduate nursing students. Dr. Jeffries has been awarded several teaching awards, including the National League for Nursing (NLN) Lucile Petry Leone Award for nursing education, the Elizabeth Russell Belford Award for teaching excellence given by Sigma Theta Tau, and numerous outstanding faculty awards presented by the graduating nursing classes. Dr. Jeffries was named project director of the 3-year NLN/Laerdal Simulation Study, a national multisite research project.

Craig A. Jones, M.D., is director of the Vermont Blueprint for Health, a program established by the state of Vermont under the leadership of its governor, legislature, and the bipartisan Health Care Reform Commission. The Blueprint is intended to guide statewide transformation of the way that health care and health services are delivered in Vermont. The program is dedicated to a high-value, high-quality health care system for all Vermonters, with a focus on prevention. Currently, Dr. Jones serves on several committees and workgroups, including the Institute of Medicine Consensus Committee on the Learning Healthcare System in America and the Roundtable on Value & Science-Driven Health Care. Before this he was an assistant professor in the Department of Pediatrics at the Keck School of Medicine at the University of Southern California and director of the

Division of Allergy/Immunology and director of the Allergy/Immunology Residency Training Program in the Department of Pediatrics at the Los Angeles County + University of Southern California Medical Center.

Patrick W. Kelley, M.D., Dr.P.H., joined the Institute of Medicine (IOM) in 2003 as director of the Board on Global Health. He has also been appointed as director of the Board on African Science Academy Development. Dr. Kelley has overseen a portfolio of IOM expert consensus studies and convened activities on subjects as wide ranging as the evaluation of the U.S. President's Emergency Plan for AIDS Relief (PEPFAR), the U.S. commitment to global health, sustainable surveillance for zoonotic infections, cardiovascular disease prevention in low- and middle-income countries, interpersonal violence prevention in low- and middle-income countries, and microbial threats to health. He also directs a unique capacity-building effort, the African Science Academy Development Initiative, which over 10 years aims to strengthen the capacity of eight African academies to provide independent, evidence-based advice to their governments on scientific matters. Prior to joining the National Academies, Dr. Kelley served in the U.S. Army for more than 23 years as a physician, residency director, epidemiologist, and program manager.

Sandeep Kishore, Ph.D., is a postdoctoral fellow at Harvard Medical School and co-chair of the Young Professionals Chronic Disease Network, a global network of 400 young professionals from 50 countries committed to the equitable prevention and treatment of noncommunicable diseases as a social justice issue. He seeks to leverage lateral thinking and transdisciplinary approaches at universities worldwide, with the goal of preparing and cultivating the next generation of young leaders to tackle health challenges of the 21st century. In this capacity he served as a delegate to the United Nations General Assembly in 2011. He is a fellow at the Massachusetts Institute of Technology Dalai Lama Center for Ethics and Transformative Values and a recipient of the Paul and Daisy Soros Fellowship for New Americans. He returned to complete his medical training at Cornell's medical college in 2012.

Maryjoan D. Ladden, Ph.D., R.N., FAAN, is a senior program officer at the Robert Wood Johnson Foundation. Her work at the foundation focuses on building a diverse and well-trained leadership and workforce in health and health care. Dr. Ladden manages most of the foundation's nursing initiatives. She leads the foundation's efforts in primary care and interprofessional collaboration. Prior to joining the foundation, she served as chief program officer of the American Nurses Association (ANA), providing strategic direction, integration, and coordination for all of ANA's programs. Dr. Ladden also spent more than 20 years as a nurse practitioner, case manager, researcher, and director of continuing professional education at Harvard

Pilgrim Health Care and as assistant professor at Harvard Medical School. Her work has focused on improving health care quality, safety, and health professional collaboration.

Lisa Lehmann, M.D., Ph.D., M.Sc., is the director of the Center for Bioethics at Brigham and Women's Hospital (BWH), associate physician in the Jen Center for Primary Care at BWH, and associate professor of medicine and medical ethics at Harvard Medical School. She joined the faculty of the Harvard Medical School Division of Medical Ethics and the BWH Division of General Internal Medicine in 1999 after completing her fellowship training in general internal medicine at Massachusetts General Hospital. Dr. Lehmann is a graduate of Cornell University and the Johns Hopkins University School of Medicine. She completed her residency training in internal medicine at Johns Hopkins Hospital and a Ph.D. in philosophy at Johns Hopkins University. She received an M.Sc. in clinical epidemiology from the Harvard School of Public Health.

Edward "Thomas" Lewis III, M.D., is a Postgraduate Year 1 psychiatry resident at the Medical University of South Carolina (MUSC) in Charleston. He graduated from MUSC in 2012 with an M.D. He also completed an interprofessional fellowship through the university. He received a B.S. in biochemistry from Queens University of Charlotte. During medical school, Dr. Lewis's extracurricular activities included being vice president of the Student Interprofessional Society and serving on the MUSC strategic planning committee for interprofessional development. He volunteered regularly at a student-run medical clinic at a local homeless shelter in town and further served as president for the campus's student psychiatry interest group.

Lorna Lynn, M.D., is the director of practice assessment development and evaluation at the American Board of Internal Medicine (ABIM). After completing a clinician–educator fellowship in general internal medicine at the University of Pennsylvania, she joined the faculty there, serving as director of ambulatory care education and winning three major teaching awards during her 8 years on the faculty. During that time she received a Robert Wood Johnson Generalist Physician Faculty Scholars Award, which funded a study of the problem faced by family caregivers of patients with HIV/AIDS. In 2000 she joined the ABIM staff, where her primary focus has been developing novel assessments as part of ABIM's program for the evaluation of clinical performance. These assessment tools, called practice improvement modules, are designed with the goal of helping physicians improve the quality of care they provide in their practices.

Lucinda L. Maine, Ph.D., serves as executive vice president and chief executive officer of the American Association of Colleges of Pharmacy (AACP). As the leading advocate for high-quality pharmacy education, AACP's vision is that academic pharmacy will work to transform the future of health care to create a world of healthy people. Dr. Maine previously served as senior vice president for policy, planning, and communications with the American Pharmacists Association (APhA). She served on the faculty at the University of Minnesota, where she practiced in the field of geriatrics, and she was an associate dean at the Samford University School of Pharmacy. Dr. Maine is a pharmacy graduate of Auburn University and received her doctorate at the University of Minnesota. Her research includes projects on aging, pharmacy manpower, and pharmacy-based immunizations. Dr. Maine has been active in leadership roles in the profession. Prior to joining the APhA staff, she served as speaker of the APhA house of delegates and as an APhA trustee. She currently serves as president of the Pharmacy Manpower Project and as a board member for Research!America.

Afaf I. Meleis, Ph.D., is the Margaret Bond Simon Dean of Nursing at the University of Pennsylvania School of Nursing, professor of nursing and sociology, and director of the school's WHO Collaborating Center for Nursing and Midwifery Leadership. Before going to Penn, she was a professor on the faculty of nursing at the University of California, Los Angeles, and at the University of California, San Francisco, for 34 years. She is a fellow of the Royal College of Nursing in the United Kingdom, the American Academy of Nursing, and the College of Physicians of Philadelphia. She is a member of the Institute of Medicine (IOM), the Robert Wood Johnson Foundation Nurse Faculty Scholar National Advisory Committee, and the George W. Bush Presidential Center Women's Initiative Policy Advisory Council; a trustee of the National Health Museum; a board member of CARE, the Josiah Macy Jr. Foundation Macy Faculty Scholars program, and the Consortium of Universities for Global Health; and chair of the IOM Global Forum on Innovation for Health Professional Education. Dr. Meleis is also president and council general emerita of the International Council on Women's Health Issues and currently serves as the global ambassador for the Girl Child Initiative of the International Council of Nurses.

Donna Meyer, R.N., M.S.N., is the dean of health sciences and project director for the Lewis and Clark Community College Family Health Clinic, a nurse-managed center. Additionally, she serves as the project director of the Lewis and Clark Family Health Clinic and mobile unit. She is currently serving as the president of the National Organization of Associate Degree Nursing. Her professional nursing activities include being a member of the Robert Wood Johnson Foundation Academic Progression in Nursing Advisory Board, the American Association of Community Colleges Affiliated Council, the Illinois Center for Nursing Advisory Board, the Illinois Healthcare Action Coalition for the Institute of Medicine/Future of Nursing, the Team Illinois/Center to Champion Nursing in America, the National Nursing Centers Consortium Health Policy Committee, and the Sigma Theta Tau International Honor Society and a site reviewer for the National League for Nursing Accrediting Commission. Dean Meyer has received various awards for her work, including the MetLife Community College Excellence Award for Innovation, the Illinois Nurses Association Innovation in Health Care Award, the Illinois Community Administrators Award for Innovation, Illinois Nursing Pinnacle Leader of the Year, the Southern Illinois University Outstanding Nursing Alumni Award, and the YWCA Woman of Distinction Award. She recently was inducted into the Southern Illinois University Hall of Fame.

J. Lloyd Michener, M.D., is professor and chair of the department of community and family medicine and director of the Duke Center for Community Research. He is a member of the board of the Association of Academic Medical Colleges, co-chair of the Community Engagement Steering Committee at the National Institutes of Health (NIH), a member of the Foundation Working Group on Public Health and Medical Education at the Centers for Disease Control and Prevention (CDC), and director of the Duke/CDC program in primary care and public health of the American Austrian Foundation–Open Medical Institute. Dr. Michener was appointed to the NIH Council for Complementary and Alternative Medicine and the Institute of Medicine Committee on Integrating Primary Care and Public Health. He was selected for membership on the newly formed National Academic Affiliations Advisory Council for the Department of Veterans Affairs and is a member of the North Carolina Institute of Medicine.

Rose Chalo Nabirye, Ph.D., M.P.H., is a senior lecturer and chair of the Department of Nursing at the School of Health Sciences, College of Health Sciences, Makerere University (MU), in Kampala, Uganda. She has been lecturing in the Department of Nursing at Makerere University since 2003 and serves on several college committees, including the School of Medicine and School of Health Sciences' institutional review boards, and graduate and research, professionalism, and mentorship committees. She is also coordinator of the Regional Master of Nursing program at MU. The program was started in collaboration with Bergen University College in Norway, the Muhimbili University of Health and Allied Sciences in Tanzania, and the University of Addis Ababa, Ethiopia. The program is funded by NORAD's Program for Master Studies. Before joining academia, she worked at

Mulago Hospital, the National Referral and Teaching Hospital in Uganda, as a registered clinical nurse and midwife for more than 20 years.

Angella Sandra Namwase is pursuing a B.S.N. at Makerere College of Health Sciences. She has great interest in women's empowerment and improved sexual and reproductive health. For this reason she created has managed to come up with an award-winning project with Make Every Woman Count, an international organization based in London. She loves to write and hopes to advocate for correction in the health system through newspaper journalism. She holds several leadership roles in her college, including as the mentorship coordinator at the undergraduate level, as the vice president of Basoga Medical Student's association, as the organizing secretary of the Students' Professionalism and Ethics Club, and as the class representative.

Warren Newton, M.D., M.P.H., serves as the vice dean of education at the University of North Carolina (UNC) School of Medicine. He is responsible for the medical students and continuing medical education. He also provides strategic direction for GME at UNC Hospitals. He has led the expansion of the UNC medical school development of a competency-based curriculum, including improving the health of populations and a new integrated clinical clerkship. Dr. Newton also serves as the William B. Aycock Distinguished Professor & Chair of Family Medicine. UNC Family Medicine has 8 campuses, 150 academic faculty, and 16 residencies and fellowships. He is an adjunct professor of epidemiology, and serves as chair of the advisory board for the Cecil G. Sheps Center for Health Services at UNC.

Sally Okun, R.N., M.M.H.S., is a member of the research, clinical, and analytics team at PatientLikeMe. As head of health data integrity and patient safety for the company, she is responsible for the site's medical ontology and the integrity of patient-reported health data. In addition, she developed and oversees the PatientsLikeMe Drug Safety and Pharmacovigilance Platform. Prior to joining PatientsLikeMe, Ms. Okun practiced as a palliative care specialist. In addition to working with patients and families facing life-changing illnesses, she was an independent consultant supporting multiyear clinical, research, and education projects focused on palliative and end-of-life care for numerous clients through Brown University, Harvard Medical School, Massachusetts Department of Mental Health, and the Robert Wood Johnson Foundation.

Scott Reeves, Ph.D., M.Sc., P.G.C.E., is the founding director of the Center for Innovation in Interprofessional Healthcare Education. He is a social scientist who has been undertaking health professions education and health services research for more than 17 years. He recently moved from Canada, where he spent the past 6 years developing conceptual, empirical, and theoretical knowledge to inform the design, implementation, and evaluation of interprofessional education and practice. He has published more than 100 peer-reviewed papers, numerous book chapters, textbooks, and monographs. He holds honorary faculty positions in a number of institutions around the world. He is also editor-in-chief of the *Journal of Interprofessional Care.*

Kathryn Rugen, Ph.D., is the nurse consultant to the Veterans Health Administration centers of excellence in primary care education. In this position she is responsible for facilitating transformation of the centers of excellence. She is also the associate chief nurse for education and research at the Jesse Brown Veterans Administration Medical Center in Chicago. Her responsibilities include nursing education and orientation, scholarship programs, nursing trainee placement, the post-baccalaureate nurse residency program, membership on the research and development committee, and chair of the collaborative institutional review board with academic affiliates (Northwestern University and University of Illinois Medical Schools). She is a practicing nurse practitioner in primary care at the Lakeside Community-based Outpatient Clinic, where she frequently acts as a preceptor to nurse practitioner students. She is an assistant professor at the University of Illinois at Chicago, College of Nursing, where she teaches research and evidence-based practice in the graduate program.

Madeline Schmitt, Ph.D., R.N., FAAN, FNAP, professor emerita, is a nurse-sociologist who, until retirement, was professor and Independence Foundation Chair in Nursing and Interprofessional Education at the University of Rochester School of Nursing. She remains active in research and publication as well as in limited teaching about interprofessional collaboration. She consults and presents nationally and internationally on the topic. Since the 1970s she has focused her career on interprofessional collaborative practice. She was a co-chair of the All Altogether, Better Health III international interprofessional education (IPE) conference in London in 2006 and the major consultant to the first American–Canadian joint conference focused on IPE—Collaborating Across Borders I—hosted in 2007 by the University of Minnesota Health Sciences Center.

Nelson Sewankambo, M.B.Ch.B., M.Sc., M.D., trained in general medicine and internal medicine at Makerere University (MU) in Uganda and later graduated with a degree in clinical epidemiology from McMaster University, Canada. He is a fellow of the Royal College of Physicians, UK, a professor of Medicine at MU, and is the principal (head) of Makerere University College of Health Sciences. Until 2007 he was dean of the Makerere University Medical School for 11 years. He contributed to the seminal work of the Sub-Saharan African Medical Schools Study (2008–2010). As co-chair of the education/production subcommittee of the Joint Learning initiative he contributed to the landmark report titled *Human Resources for Health: Overcoming the Crisis*, which had a major influence on the WHO and its subsequent 2006 report, *Together for Health*, which focused on the global crisis of health workers and the need for urgent action to enhance population health.

Stefanus Snyman, M.B.Ch.B., DOM, is the manager of interprofessional education and service-learning at the Centre for Health Professions Education, Faculty of Medicine and Health Sciences, Stellenbosch University, South Africa. He is a qualified occupational medicine practitioner and health professions educationalist. His special interest is interprofessional practice and how it strengthens health systems and improves patient outcomes. He is a member of the Functioning and Disability Work Group of the World Health Organization, advising on issues related to health professions education and e-learning.

Elizabeth Speakman, Ed.D., R.N., is co-director of the Jefferson Center for Interprofessional Education and associate professor of nursing at Thomas Jefferson University. Since joining the university in 2003, Dr. Speakman has served as assistant dean of the R.N.-to-B.S.N. program and, most recently, as associate dean for student affairs. She is principal investigator on the Robert Wood Johnson Foundation New Careers in Nursing grant, which to date has funded $430,000 in scholarships for second-degree nursing students enrolled in the one-year facilitated accelerated course track program. Recognition of Dr. Speakman's leadership role in nursing education includes fellowship in the Academy of Nursing Education, selection as a Johnson & Johnson and a Jonas Foundation Faculty Mentor, and a Robert Wood Johnson Foundation Executive Nurse Fellow.

Harrison C. Spencer, M.D., M.P.H., became the first full-time president and chief executive officer of the Association of Schools and Programs of Public Health in 2000. From 1996 to 2000, Dr. Spencer was dean of the London School of Hygiene and Tropical Medicine. Before then he was dean of the Tulane School of Public Health and Tropical Medicine in New Orleans. During his career with the Centers for Disease Control and Prevention (CDC), Dr. Spencer served as an Epidemic Intelligence Service officer and at the field station in El Salvador. He founded and for 5 years (1979–1984) directed the CDC research station in Nairobi, Kenya, and he then served as senior medical officer at the World Health Organization Malaria Action

Program in Geneva. Dr. Spencer was elected a founding fellow of the UK Academy of Medical Sciences in 1998 and to the Institute of Medicine in 2003.

Maria Tassone, M.Sc., is the inaugural director of the Centre for Interprofessional Education, a strategic partnership between the University of Toronto and the University Health Network (UHN). She is also the senior director of health professions and interprofessional care and integration at the UHN in Toronto, a network of four hospitals: Toronto General, Toronto Western, Toronto Rehab, and Princess Margaret. Ms. Tassone holds a B.S. in physical therapy from McGill University and an M.S. from the University of Western Ontario, and she is an assistant professor in the department of physical therapy, Faculty of Medicine, University of Toronto. Ms. Tassone was the UHN project lead for the coaching arm of the Catalyzing and Sustaining Communities of Collaboration Around Interprofessional Care, which was recently awarded the Ontario Hospital Association international Ted Freedman Award for Education Innovation.

John Tegzes, M.A., V.M.D., has an educational and professional background that includes nursing, psychology, and veterinary medicine. He has worked as a nurse primarily in community health and hospice and as a veterinarian in small animal practice. He is a board-certified specialist in clinical toxicology, and he has worked for the California Poison Control System, the Oregon Poison Center, and a state diagnostic toxicology laboratory. Currently he serves as the director of interprofessional education at the Western University of Health Sciences with a joint appointment as a professor of toxicology. His work at Western focuses primarily on preparing graduates from nine health professions for collaborative, team-based practice.

George E. Thibault, M.D., became the seventh president of the Josiah Macy Jr. Foundation in 2008. Immediately prior to that, he served as vice president of clinical affairs at Partners Healthcare System in Boston and as director of the academy at Harvard Medical School (HMS). He was the first Daniel D. Federman Professor of Medicine and Medical Education at HMS and is now the Federman Professor, Emeritus. Dr. Thibault previously served as chief medical officer at Brigham and Women's Hospital and as chief of medicine at the Harvard-affiliated Brockton/West Roxbury Veterans Administration Hospital. He was associate chief of medicine and director of the internal medical residency program at the Massachusetts General Hospital (MGH). At the MGH he also served as director of the Medical Intensive Care Unit and as founding director of the Medical Practice Evaluation Unit.

Samuel O. Thier, M.D., is professor of medicine and health care policy emeritus at Harvard Medical School. He had been a professor of medicine in those areas at Harvard Medical School from 1994 to 2007. Previously he served as president and chief executive officer of Partners HealthCare System, president of Massachusetts General Hospital, and president of Brandeis University. He served as president of the Institute of Medicine and as chair of the department of internal medicine at Yale University School of Medicine, where he was Sterling Professor. Dr. Thier is a director of Charles River Laboratories, Inc., and the Foundation of the National Institutes of Health. He is a member of the board of overseers of Cornell University Weill Medical College, the board of overseers of Brandeis University Heller School for Social Policy and Management (chair), and the board of dean's advisors of Harvard School of Public Health.

Brigid Vaughan, M.D., attended New York Medical College and Robert Wood Johnson Medical School, then trained in child and adolescent psychiatry at New Jersey Medical School and Children's Hospital Boston (CHB)/Harvard Medical School. She worked at CHB for more than 15 years. Early on she was medical director of inpatient psychiatry, and later she served in an outpatient role, specializing in the treatment of substance use disorders. She was co-founder of the Adolescent Substance Abuse Program, served as its first director of psychiatry and as clinical associate with the Center for Adolescent Substance Abuse Research, and became the director of psychopharmacology at Children's.

Sarita Verma, L.L.B., M.D., is a professor in the Department of Family and Community Medicine, deputy dean of the Faculty of Medicine, and associate vice provost for health professions education at the University of Toronto (U of T). She has been a diplomat in Canada's foreign service and worked with the Office of the United Nations High Commissioner for Refugees in Sudan and Ethiopia for several years. Dr. Verma is the 2006 recipient of the Donald Richards Wilson Award in medical education from the Royal College of Physicians and Surgeons of Canada and the 2009 corecipient of the May Cohen Gender Equity Award from the Association of Faculties of Medicine in Canada. Along with colleagues at McGill University, the University of British Columbia, and U of T she has been the lead consultant for the Future of Medical Education in Canada–Postgraduate project on the Liaison and Engagement Strategy and the Environmental Scan Scientific Study. As deputy dean, Dr. Verma leads strategic planning and implementation as well as communications and external relations. Additionally, she is responsible for integrated education across the health sciences and liaison with affiliated partners.

Patricia Hinton Walker, Ph.D., R.N., has held national prominence for more than 25 years as a leader in health care and health sciences education as the dean of a school of nursing. She is a Chief Nursing Officer in hospital- and community-based care and in the health information technology and policy arenas. She serves as senior advisor to the TIGER (Technology Informatics Guiding Education Reform) Initiative Foundation and is often sought to speak on topics such as health informatics; the use of technology in education, practice, and research; leadership; and cultural change in health care and education. She is currently vice president for policy and strategic initiatives at the Uniformed Services University of the Health Sciences, where she previously served as dean. In 2001 she was senior scholar in residence at the Agency for Healthcare Research and Policy, focusing on cost and quality outcomes as well as on patient safety research. Currently she serves as an internal coach and consultant on patient safety and TeamSTEPPS to the DoD (Department of Defense) Patient Safety Program within Tricare Management Activity (a component of the Military Health Care System).

Margaretha Wilhelmsson, Ph.D., is a biomedical scientist. She worked in hospital laboratories and with blood banks for many years before she became a lecturer and vice study director in the education of biomedical scientists at Linköping University. For more than 20 years Dr. Wilhelmsson has been involved in the interprofessional education program in Linköping, called "The Linköping model," both as a tutor and as a director of study. Dr. Wilhelmsson's research focuses on interprofessional competence. A central question she has sought to answer is "Can interprofessional competence be trained?"

Jenny Wong is a third-year pharmacy student at the University of Minnesota. She is currently the chair of CLARION, a student-driven, staff- and faculty-advised committee focused on co-curricular, interprofessional experiences for University of Minnesota Academic Health Center students. CLARION holds a yearly national case-based competition in which interprofessional teams of students present a root cause analysis of a fictitious sentinel event to a panel of senior-level health executives. She graduated from the University of North Carolina at Chapel Hill with a bachelor's degree in information science and public health and previously worked as a consultant in Washington, DC.

Paul Worley, MBBS, Ph.D., is dean of medicine at Flinders University in Adelaide, Australia. Dr. Worley studied medicine at the University of Adelaide. In 1992 he was elected president of the Rural Doctors Association of South Australia, and in 1994 he was appointed senior lecturer in rural health at Flinders University. In addition to maintaining an active clinical workload in rural and urban practice, he is responsible for coordinating the rapid expansion of Flinders University's rural programs. He is also the past academic director on the board of the Australian College of Rural and Remote Medicine and the executive chair of the Rural and Remote Area Placement Program. In 2001 Dr. Worley was appointed professor and director of the Flinders University Rural Clinical School and editor-in-chief of *Rural and Remote Health*, the international journal of rural and remote health research, education, practice, and policy.

Matthew K. Wynia, M.D., M.P.H., is an internist and specialist in infectious diseases. At the American Medical Association he oversees projects on topics that include learning from medical errors, physician professionalism, ethics and epidemics, medicine and the Holocaust, and inequities in health and health care. Dr. Wynia is the author of more than 125 published articles and a book on fairness in health care benefit design. His work has been published in leading medical and health policy journals, and he has been a guest on *ABC News Nightline*, the BBC World Service, NPR, and other programs. Dr. Wynia cares for patients at the University of Chicago.

Brenda Zierler, Ph.D., R.N., conducts research exploring the relationships between the delivery of health care and outcomes at both the patient and system level. Her primary appointment is in the School of Nursing at the University of Washington, but she holds three adjunct appointments: two in the School of Medicine (department of surgery and department of medical education and biomedical informatics), and one in the School of Public Health (department of health services). As co–principal investigator of a Josiah Macy Jr. Foundation–funded study (with Brian Ross, M.D., Ph.D.), Dr. Zierler leads a group of interprofessional faculty and students in the development of a simulation-based, team training program to improve collaborative interprofessional communication both within teams and with patients. Her team is currently validating the impact of simulation-based team training on students' interprofessional communication skills as measured by an innovative Web-based assessment tool.

Sanjay P. Zodpey, M.D., Ph.D., works as director of public health education at the Public Health Foundation of India (PHFI), New Delhi, and also holds a leadership role as director at Indian Institutes of Public Health, Delhi. He served as director of Indian Institute of Public Health, Gandhinagar and Bhubaneswar. He earlier worked as professor of preventive and social medicine and as vice dean at Government Medical College, Nagpur. Professor Zodpey is involved in designing several capacity development initiatives, including long-term academic programs at PHFI. He is currently undertaking situation analysis of education for health professions in India. He is also involved in several research initiatives related to education for health professionals, including designing competency-based frameworks for various categories of health professionals; the assessment of the impact of educational initiatives on performance of health professionals; research in the governance of education for health professionals in India; and estimation of the need of various categories of health professionals in the country. He is currently leading the project supported by the U.S. Agency for International Development for designing human resources for health policy for the government of Jharkhand (India).

C

Summary of Updates Provided by Members of the Global Forum on Innovation in Health Professional Education's Innovation Collaboratives

The Institute of Medicine's (IOM's) Global Forum on Innovation in Health Professional Education is complemented by the work of four university- or foundation-based collaborations in Canada, India, South Africa, and Uganda. Known as innovation collaboratives (ICs), these country-based collaborations characterize innovators in health professional education through their demonstration projects on how schools of nursing, public health, and medicine can work together toward a common goal. The four ICs were selected by IOM leadership through a competitive application process that provides for certain benefits on the Forum. These benefits include

- the appointment of one innovation collaborative representative to the IOM Global Forum;
- time on each workshop agenda to showcase and discuss the IC's project with leading health interprofessional educators and funding organizations;
- written documentation of each collaborative's progress summarized in the Global Forum workshop reports published by the National Academies Press; and
- remote participation in Global Forum workshops through a video feed to the collaborative's home site.

Each collaborative is undertaking a different 2-year program of innovative curricular and institutional development that specifically responds to one of the recommendations in the Lancet Commission or the 2011 IOM *The Future of Nursing* report—reports that inspired the establishment of the Global Forum. These on-the-ground innovations involve a substantial and coordinated effort among at least the three partnered schools (a medical school, a nursing school, and a public health school). As ad hoc activities of the Global Forum, the innovation collaboratives are amplifying the process of revaluating health professional education globally so that it can be done more efficiently and more effectively and so that it will create increased capacity for task sharing, teamwork, and health systems leadership. The work of each of the collaboratives is detailed below.

CANADA

Maria Tassone, M.Sc., B.Sc.PT
Sarita Verma, LLB, M.D., CCFP
University of Toronto

The Canadian Interprofessional Health Leadership Collaborative

The Canadian Interprofessional Health Leadership Collaborative (CIHLC) is a multi-institutional and interprofessional partnership that includes the faculties and schools of medicine, nursing, and public health and the programs of interprofessional education (IPE) at five universities. The collaborative, led by the University of Toronto, also contains the University of British Columbia, the Northern Ontario School of Medicine, Queen's University, and Université Laval as regional leads, as well as these institutions' affiliated networks with multiple sites in Canada, the United States, and the rest of the world (see Figure C-1). The goal of the CIHLC is to develop, implement, evaluate, and disseminate an evidence-based program for collaborative leadership in five phases over the next 3 years. The education program will be targeted to health care leaders, practitioners, and students.

The first phase of the project included the identification of university leads, recruitment of staff, and the establishment of a national steering committee (NSC) and a secretariat to steer and support the project. The NSC has representation from each of the five universities. Through weekly telephone meetings, the leads, alternates, and research associates have been building synergies while delving into questions and discussion around the meaning of key project components. These have included defining what is meant by "collaborative leadership," "collaborative leadership curriculum," "community engagement," "social accountability," and "social responsibility," as well as exploring early ideas about evaluation frameworks for the program and project.

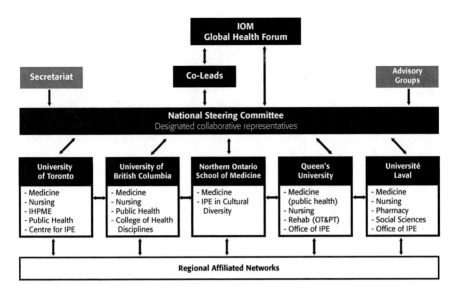

FIGURE C-1 CIHLC structure.
SOURCE: CIHLC.

A CIHLC engagement plan calls for early engagement of stakeholders and communities to ensure successful uptake and support for the project. As such, the CIHLC leads have been building partnerships within their own universities which represent multiple health sciences faculties. They have also been using their established provincial and regional networks within Canada to inform and receive input on the CIHLC project and the potential opportunities provided by membership on the IOM Global Forum on Innovation in Health Professional Education. From a knowledge translation and scholarship perspective, the partners have presented this information at several relevant conferences and presented posters on the project at two international conferences in Thunder Bay, Canada, and Kobe, Japan, in October 2012. CIHLC partners have also been using their networks to stimulate discussion about the Lancet report and how recommendations could be applied to Canadian health education reform.

The second phase, which is aimed at knowledge acquisition, is under way, by way of planning for and implementing phased literature reviews to identify what has been done in the peer-reviewed and grey literature and to identify gaps that have already begun to refine the objectives of the project. Several literature reviews are in various stages of implementation and are leading the evolution of the CIHLC program and its key components. Those key components are the definition and impact of collaborative leadership for health system change, the existing evidence base for collaborative leadership education, the principles of community engagement and social accountability, and the validity of potential evaluation frameworks.

The first literature review that will serve as the foundation for the project has been completed. It was intended to establish the level and rigor of evidence related to collaborative leadership for health system change and, ultimately, to identify what type of collaborative leadership best enables the global transformation of the health care system. Once the broad framework for the literature review had been established, attention turned to scholarly search engines. Initial search terms included "health care leadership," "collaborative leadership," "collaborative leadership" AND "healthcare," "change leadership healthcare," and "change management healthcare." Initial databases consulted included Google Scholar, the Summon multidisciplinary search engine at the University of Toronto, PubMed Health, Longwoods Publishing, and ProQuest. It became clear very early that the search strategy required targeting because the initial search on the term "collaborative leadership," limited to scholarly journals in Summon, turned up more than 72,000 hits.

With the basic field this enormous, the CIHLC's working description of the "future collaborative change leader" was used as context and as a filter for the review. In total, 183 journal articles or reports and approximately two dozen theoretical books were reviewed. From this, it was clear that "collaborative leadership" is less a definable concept and that assessing the evidence is difficult because there is no single entity, model, or framework that leads to one definition. At this stage the literature review has led the project team to note that while the term "collaborative leadership" is applied to diverse ways of practicing collaboration, it is generally aimed at the broad movement away from an "individual expert" model of leadership to drawing on multiple perspectives for richer responses to complex questions or needs. This movement from individual experts is broadly described as a necessity in a world of increasing complexity and rapid change, where no one person or perspective could possibly comprehend or influence the kinds of responses, thinking, and actions required for sustainability.

Within this basic, shared perspective, the concept of "collaborative leadership" covers a huge range of discussions. At one end of the range, the concept is used to describe leaders with positional authority who are learning to share power and decision making in different ways but who are not fundamentally changing traditional models of organization and structure. This literature tends to continue to focus on leaders as individuals. The term is also applied in various ways to the actions required to enable collaborative action within and across systems, whether from formal leaders or among group members.

The CIHLC's current definition of collaborative leadership is as follows:

> Collaborative leadership is a way of being, reflected in attitudes, behaviours, and actions that are enabled by individuals, teams, and/or organizations and integrated within and across complex adaptive systems to transform health with people and communities, locally and globally.

With the first literature review completed, the collaborative is now engaged in further refinement and validation on the definition of "collaborative leadership" for health system change. Qualitative research is being undertaken through key informant interviews with up to 30 people. The subjects will include senior leaders in IPE; Canadian educators; government, hospital and student leaders; and international thought leaders. The results of this qualitative research, along with the literature review, will inform the leadership curriculum work that is under way.

A systematic literature review of existing curricula in interprofessional collaborative leadership has been launched. Review questions have been formulated, key concepts have been identified, a search strategy format for key databases has been identified, and the search strategy has been tested for efficiency and effectiveness of journal article retrieval. The literature review will assess the impacts of leadership curricula on health care practices and on skills, attitudes, and behaviors of learners at pre-qualification, post-qualification, and executive levels. It will also inform which leadership competencies are addressed in existing curricula and what pedagogical methods are used. Based on the results, the CIHLC will adopt or adapt an existing leadership curriculum or else will develop something new. Ultimately, the goal is to produce a template or toolkit of collaborative leadership curriculums that will be culturally validated in both French and English languages and will be pilot tested among different groups of learners across Canada.

At the same time, an evaluation framework is being developed that will include measurement indicators for systematic implementation. This product will support the pilot testing of the collaborative leadership curriculum. The CIHLC is also conducting a literature review of community engagement principles that includes an understanding of the competencies that underlie social responsibility and the principles that collaborative leaders should apply in their own or their organization's social accountability.

The work thus far confirms that the CIHLC's initial model for the "future collaborative change leader" is consistent with the emerging focus on the need for health system influencers to be able to take meaningful action and to inspire positive movement in a world of multiple perspectives, ambiguity, and intricacy. The emphases in our emerging model on transformation, complexity, adaptation, learning, and distributive leadership all convey a context of transformative, systemic change. Our program will need to focus on the kind of leader who enables a more sustainable, equitable, fair, and just way of harnessing existing resources and the creation of meaningful innovation across all health professions.

INDIA

Sanjay Zodpey, M.D., Ph.D.
Public Health Institute of India

Building Interdisciplinary Leadership Skills Among Health Professionals in the 21st Century: An Innovative Training Model

Rationale for the Initiative

Health professionals have made enormous contributions globally to health and development during the past century; complacency will only continue the ineffective application of 20th-century educational strategies that are unfit to tackle 21st-century challenges. The demand of 21st-century health professional education is mainly transformational, aiming to help the professionals strategically identify emerging health challenges and innovatively address the needs of the population. As in many other countries, the need of the hour in India is to amalgamate the skills and knowledge of the medical, nursing, and public health professionals and to develop robust leadership competencies among them. This initiative proposes to identify the interdisciplinary leadership competencies among doctors, nurses and public health experts that are necessary to bring about a positive change in the health care system of the country. Once they are identified, an interdisciplinary training model will be conceptualized and piloted with an objective to develop these leadership competencies and skills among the various health care professionals.

Objectives of the Initiative

1. Identification of interdisciplinary health care leadership competencies relevant to the medical, nursing, and public health professional education in India.
2. Conceptualization of and piloting an interprofessional training model to develop physician, nursing, and public health leadership skills relevant for the 21st-century health system in India.

Partners of the Proposed Regional Innovation Collaborative

The proposed Regional Innovation Collaborative will be a partnership among three schools: the Public Health Foundation of India, New Delhi (public health institute); the Datta Meghe Institute of Medical Sciences, Sawangi (medical school); and the Symbiosis College of Nursing, Pune (nursing school). These schools will team up to further the objective of the collaborative.

Proposed Workplan

The three partner institutes will collaborate to address the major objectives of this initiative. The following activities, in chronological order, are proposed by the Regional Innovation Collaborative as part of the workplan following a formal approval of the proposal by the IOM:

1. **Constitution of the collaborative:** A team will be formed that includes members from all three partner institutes. The national program lead will represent the collaborative as a member of the Global Forum at the headquarters of the IOM.

2. **Constitution of a Technical Advisory Group (TAG):** The TAG will consist of renowned experts in the field of health professions education. The mandate of this group will be to oversee and provide guidance to the activities of the collaborative. The TAG will meet once in every 6 months to review the progress of the collaborative's work and to discuss the further steps to be taken under the initiative.

3. **Identification of interdisciplinary health care leadership competencies:** The initial activities to be undertaken by the collaborative would include an exhaustive literature search by the working group under the guidance of the program leads to understand the need for and genesis of leadership competencies as a part of education of health professionals. Published evidence, both global and Indian, shall be included in the literature search to look for key interdisciplinary leadership competencies, the need for an interdisciplinary training of health professionals, and the current scenarios in interprofessional health education. The literature search strategies will include the searching of journal articles from electronic databases, medical journals, grey literature, newspaper articles, and papers presented in conferences.

A sensitive electronic search strategy will be used to locate the articles in Medline as well as other databases. The search will not be restricted by the period of publication or language. The electronic search will be complemented by hand searching for relevant publications and documents in their bibliographies. A process of snowballing will be used until no new articles are located.

The Public Health Foundation of India (PHFI) is currently undertaking a project in India as part of the 5-C Network. Within this regional network of five countries in Southeast Asia, PHFI is involved in a situational analysis of the medical, nursing, and public health professions at a national level. The aim of this activity is to conduct a landscaping exercise to understand the current situation in these disciplines with regard to issues such as governance, policy, and challenges encountered. As part of the situational analysis, PHFI will also carry out an institutional level assessment and evaluate the instructional processes being followed in these streams. Additionally, a graduate survey will be carried out with participation of current students as well as alumni in order to understand the framework of competencies. The findings of this national assessment will also be incorporated into the literature search activity.

The collaborative shall hold regular meetings with participation from all three partner institutes. During these meetings, the group shall deliberate on the findings of the initial literature search and align the proposed activities within the broader context of the objectives of the collaborative. The proposed duration for this activity is 6 months.

4. Expert group meetings: Once the literature search is complete, the working group will summarize the findings of the search and prepare a formal report. The summary report will be circulated for detailed review by the senior members of the collaborative. The TAG will also review the report and guide the findings. Once the report and its findings are finalized, these will be shared with the Global Forum of the IOM. The duration for this activity will be 3 months.

5. Consultation: The next activity under the collaborative will be a consultation with experts from various disciplines of health professional education where the findings of the literature search will be presented. This would be a 2-day meeting in New Delhi hosted by PHFI and its partners. The agenda of the consultation would focus on the leadership issues in the fields of medicine, nursing, and public health in India. The agenda will include a discussion of the current situation in the fields of medical, nursing, and public health leadership in India, followed by a presentation of the findings of the literature search. The second half of the agenda for the consultation would be devoted to group presentations where the expert group will deliberate on the strategies for the development of a standardized leadership competency framework for interprofessional health education across identified streams of health professionals.

The proposed experts would include the following: representatives from various Indian institutions, such as the Ministry of Health and Family Welfare, the Indian Council of Medical Research, the Medical Council of India, the Indian Nursing Council, the National Board of Examinations, and the University Grants Commission; representatives from agencies such as the World Health Organization; academics from premier public health schools in India; and senior officials from associations such as the Indian Association of Preventive and Social Medicine (IAPSM), the Indian Public Health Association (IPHA), and the Indian Medical Association (IMA). They will all be invited to the 2-day consultation.

The suggestions and recommendations of the consultation shall be incorporated by the collaborative's partner institutes to line up with the objectives. This will also form the basis for planning and piloting the interprofessional training model for physicians, nurses, and public health personnel.

The proposed duration for this activity, including the groundwork for the consultation, its conduction, and the preparation of the report, would be 3 months.

6. *Developing a training model*: The next activity of the project will be the development of the training model for the pilot. Based on the findings of the literature search and the recommendations of the expert group at the consultation, a training model will be conceptualized. The design of this model will integrate the leadership skills of all three disciplines and will be adapted to suit the Indian health system scenario.

A training manual will be developed for use in the trainings by the working group along with the team leaders. The training manual will incorporate suggestions from TAG members as well.

Learning objectives: At the end of the training, the participants would

- Have an understanding of transformative learning, including the importance of health care leadership in the 21st century and the interdependence of health care education among health professionals for the development of change agents.
- Be trained to understand the application of leadership competencies in their local health care settings.
- Have an understanding of how the application of these competencies would help them to tackle emerging health care challenges in their local health care settings.

The training will be targeted at in-service professionals across the country from the medical, nursing, and public health fields as well as students in these streams. Inculcating interdisciplinary leadership skills among medical, nursing, and public health students will aim at transforming them into change agents at an early stage in their careers. The long-term objective of this training model would be its integration into the regular curriculum of the medical, nursing, and public health students with an aim to develop interdisciplinary leadership skills among them. The trainers will be faculty members from medical and nursing colleges and public health institutes. To achieve this goal, we will advocate the importance of this model through various national associations such as IAPSM, IPHA, etc. It is proposed that the training model will be implemented with the support of the state governments as well as of the central government.

Before the trainings are implemented at various sites, this model will be pilot tested on some in-service professionals and students across the three streams. For this, a detailed agenda and the training material will be prepared based on the content of the training manual.

7. Piloting the training model:

Participants—The pilot trainings will be conducted in four batches. For the first two batches the target group will be in-service doctors, nurses, and public health personnel from health care centers in and around New Delhi, Sawangi, and Pune. These would be personnel working at district hospitals, community health centers, private clinics and hospitals, and primary health centers. The size of the group for each training workshop will be about 15 to 20, with approximately 6 to 7 trainees from each stream.

The next two batches will train students from all three disciplines. The number of trainees for each batch of students will be 15 to 20, with 6 to 7 students from each stream. The pilot model would, thus, aim to train approximately 30 to 40 in-service candidates and about 30 to 40 students belonging to medical, nursing, and public health professions.

Trainers—Resource faculty from the three partner institutes as well as experts from other organizations, such as the Ministry of Health and Family Welfare, the World Health Organization, academia (professors from the community medicine department at medical colleges), and professional medical, nursing and public health bodies, will be invited to participate as trainers and guest faculty.

Contents and duration of the training—The proposed duration of the training is three days. This pilot training workshop will include both didactic sessions and group discussions. The didactic sessions will aim at giving the trainees an understanding of leadership skills and their importance in health care. The aim of the group discussions will be to train the trainees to innovatively apply interdisciplinary leadership competencies in their local health care settings.

The first day of the training would focus on giving the trainees an overview of the concept of interdisciplinary leadership among health professionals. This would be through didactic lectures. The trainees would also be given an opportunity to work in groups during the second half of the day and to present their views on the same. The second day of the training would focus on how these leadership skills can be applied by these professionals in their own local health care settings. One to two didactic sessions will be followed by a group presentation on day 2 as well. The third day will consist of open sessions in which the trainees will have an opportunity to interact with the faculty and to give feedback about the training and will be evaluated on the basis of participation in group discussion, presentations, and interaction.

All four batches of pilot training will be conducted out of the three partner institutes. At the end of each training workshop, a formal report will be prepared and shared with the concerned stakeholders. The trainees will also be asked to fill out a feedback form, the responses to which will be incorporated in the report. Based on the feedback and the experience of each training workshop, certain amendments may be made to the subsequent trainings to incorporate the suggestions. The pilot trainings will be conducted over a 6-month period.

8. Preparation and dissemination of findings: At the end of the pilot phase of training, a detailed final report will be prepared by members of the collaborative with inputs from the TAG. This report, in addition to interim reports about each activity, will be shared with all concerned national and international key stakeholders. The findings of the initiative will be published as a monograph and also in peer-reviewed journal. The collaborative will also present the findings of the initiative to the Global Forum on Health Professional Education.

Parallel to the activities of the collaborative as part of this initiative, the national program lead will represent the collaborative in the semi-annual workshops of the IOM and will present the ongoing work of the collaborative to initiate discussion among global stakeholders and receive inputs and suggestions from the entire Global Forum community.

Funding Support

The Indian Council of Medical Research will be approached for funding for this 2-year activity.

SOUTH AFRICA

Marietjie de Villiers, Ph.D., M.B.Ch.B., M.Fam.Med.
Stefanus Snyman, M.B.Ch.B., DOM
Stellenbosch University

South African Partnership on Innovation in Health Professional Education

The South African collaborative involves Stellenbosch University, the University of the Western Cape, and the University of the Free State collaborating on two overlapping yet distinct projects in innovation in health professional education.

Project 1: To identify the relevant competencies required for transformational and shared leadership and design and to implement a suitable leadership program for health teams.

The focus of this project is on leadership capacity building of health professional educators and young professionals. The principles of interdependence and transformative learning underpin the framework proposed by Frenk et al. (2010). In the proposed reforms that will result in interdependence and transformative learning there is a recurring theme of leadership. This is anchored in the argument that transformative learning is about developing leadership attributes in order to produce enlightened change agents, which is then explicitly or implicitly woven into all the proposed instructional and institutional reforms. Leadership is therefore no longer the domain of the organizational leaders, but is shared. To optimize the potential for success of these reforms, the focus should be not only on the training of the new professionals, but also, especially in the initial stages, on capacity building of the existing teaching staff and practicing professionals, especially since role modeling is regarded as an integral part of the success (Interprofessional Education Collaborative Expert Panel, 2011).

Components of the Project

1. Determine the leadership competencies that are valued as important and relevant in an interprofessional, multicultural environment, framed in the transformational (Bass, 1990), empowering (Albrecht and Andreetta, 2011), and shared leadership (Pearce et al., 2009) paradigms, also exploring aspects of positive (Cameron, 2008) and strengths-based (Rath and Conchie, 2008) leadership and positioned within the concept of cultural dimensions (Hofstede, 2010).

2. Design an interprofessional leadership competency framework.
3. Develop and implement:
   a. A leadership training programme with a multi-institutional, interprofessional, team-based approach initially at the level of professional educators and young qualified professionals. This will take an interprofessional team-based approach.
   b. Appropriate assessment and evaluation tools.
   c. A system of continued and sustained support and development.

Project 2: To design and implement competency-based interprofessional skills building for teamwork in community and primary health care settings.

The aim of this project is to develop effective interprofessional collaboration competencies in students and educators. It will contribute to the development of social accountability in graduates, institutional partners, and primary health care services. The patient- and community-centered approach of the project will foster interprofessional teamwork and also assist with restructuring health professions curricula in response to the health needs of society (Frenk et al., 2010; de Villiers and Naidoo, 2011).

The collaboration between the various IPE units at the Faculty of Health Sciences, the Boland Nursing College in Worcester, and the University of the Western Cape Faculty of Community and Health Sciences' School of Nursing was started in 2010 by placing students together in community service learning projects. This IAP teamwork project was born out of these efforts. Encouraging progress has already been made in developing mobile applications for household and health systems surveys in a rural setting.

Interprofessional training workshops with primary health care professionals and community workers to strengthen patient- and community-centered care have also been conducted. This was further supported by the installation of video link facilities at rural clinical training sites.

This project is designed to

1. Facilitate and coordinate appropriate curriculum renewal processes aiming to integrate interprofessional teamwork competencies longitudinally throughout the curricula. These renewals could include, inter alia, signature leaning experiences at the beginning of the first year with student involvement in household and health systems surveys in a rural community, in partnership with local communities. In consequent years IPE service learning activities will be developed using relevant interactive communicative technology approaches and equipment.

2. Develop an innovative formative and summative assessment model to longitudinally evaluate the development of teamwork competencies.
3. Build capacity for effective patient- and community-centered role models in interprofessional teamwork, in both a clinical and community setting, among lecturers, clinical supervisors, and community partners (Interprofessional Education Collaborative Expert Panel, 2011).
4. Design and implement an appropriate evaluation of the above three areas to identify the good practice models, challenges, and opportunities for such curriculum renewal processes for IPE.

UGANDA

Rose Chalo Nabirye, Ph.D., M.P.H.
Nelson Sewankambo, M.B.Ch.B., M.Sc., M.D., F.R.C.P., L.L.D. (HC)
Makerere University

Defining competencies, developing and implementing an interprofessional training model to develop competencies and skills in the realm of health professions ethics and professionalism

Innovation and Motivation for Selection of Innovation

This project is a major innovation aimed at contributing to improvement in the quality of health service. Although there is a lot of discussion about the need to improve professional ethics and professionalism in low- and middle-income countries, there has been very little attempt to develop competence-based interprofessional education programs to address the challenges. Professionalism is defined in several different ways (Wilkinson et al., 2009). The Royal College of Physicians (2005) has defined professionalism as "a set of values, behaviors, and relationships that underpin the trust the public has in doctors." This definition can be extended to embrace all types of health workers.

Overall Aim: To prepare a future workforce committed to practicing to a high degree of ethics and professionalism and performing effectively as part of an interprofessional health team with leadership skills.

Specific Objectives

1. To define competencies and develop a curriculum for interprofessional education of health professional students (nursing, medicine,

public health, dentistry, pharmacy, and radiography) in order to develop their skills in the realm of ethics and professionalism.

2. To pilot a curriculum for interprofessional education of health professional students (nursing, medicine, public health, dentistry, pharmacy, and radiography) to develop their skills in the realm of ethics and professionalism.

3. To develop curriculum for interprofessional education for health workers and tutors in ethics and professionalism and pilot its implementation in partnership with the regulatory professional councils.

Approach to Implementation of the Project

Instructional Reforms

A critical element of this project will be the engagement of major stakeholders, including the Ministry of Health, patients, hospitals and health centers, private practitioners, professional councils, educators, students, alumni, and consumer rights groups nationally. This engagement will ensure the participation of stakeholders in the implementation and the commitment of local resources to support this effort. Through this engagement the collaborative will define the extent of the problem (unethical and unprofessional practices among nurses, doctors, public health workers, and other health professionals) and identify the necessary interventions, including the required competences and interprofessional training approaches that will address the gaps as well as the necessary post-training support to ensure the institutionalization of ethics and professionalism among health professionals in Uganda. Stakeholders will participate in the implementation of training and mentoring trainees at their respective places of work. Of particular importance are the students who have initiated the formation of a student ethics and professionalism club. They are advanced in the planning process and will be supported through this project and contribute to the whole process of this project. Right from the beginning, the collaborative plans to align this educational project with the needs of Uganda's population. Concerns have been raised about ethics and professionalism among health professionals in Uganda, largely by the media. There are, however, only limited brief reports in publications in the recent past in peer-reviewed literature on the issue of ethics and professionalism among health workers in Uganda (Hagopian et al., 2009; Kiguli et al., 2011; Kizza et al., 2011).

Some national reports highlight the challenges in this area, but few formal studies have been conducted to document the extent of the problem, the contextual factors and possible interventions (UNHCO, 2003, 2010).

Because of the lack of comprehensive evaluations and evidence the collaborative plans to initiate this project with a systematic needs assessment. The needs assessment will involve the participation of representatives from several key partners mentioned previously. Data will be collected through an analysis of key documents from the professional councils, which are statutory units charged with the responsibility of investigating reports and cases of professional indiscipline among doctors, dentists, nurses, pharmacists, and others. The collaborative shall undertake limited surveys and key informant interviews among the above-named groups.

Development and Implementation of the Curriculum

Results from the needs assessments will be used to inform the curriculum development process, which will employ the six-step approach (Kern et al., 2009). Prior to curriculum development, interprofessional competencies will be defined through stakeholder engagement and suggestions, building on the five competencies defined by the 2003 IOM report *Health Professions Education: A Bridge to Quality*. Trainees will learn not only competencies related to ethical practices and professionalism but also competencies of interprofessional collaboration and leadership (Interprofessional Education Collaborative Expert Panel, 2011). Stakeholder discussions will be held to get a clearer understanding of society's needs and the challenges of ensuring high standards of ethics and professionalism. This will be followed by a consensus process to arrive at an agreed-upon set of competencies to be acquired during an interdisciplinary course for the students who are the next generation of leaders.

A curriculum will be developed for students and for teachers based on the needs assessment results and the defined competencies.

Institutional Reforms

A number of institutional reforms will be needed as the instructional reforms are implemented. These include a careful review of the linkages and collaboration between the university and the aforementioned stakeholders, and the recognition and the reward system for excellence in demonstrating the desired high standards of ethics and professionalism among both students and staff.

REFERENCES

Albrecht, S., and M. Andreetta. 2011. The influence of empowering leadership, empowerment and engagement on affective commitment and turnover intentions in community health service workers: Test of a model. *Leadership in Health Services* 24(3):228–237.

Bass, B. M. 1990. From transactional to transformational leadership: Learning to share the vision. *Organizational Dynamics* 18(3):19–31.

Cameron, K. 2008. *Positive leadership: Strategies for extraordinary performance.* San Francisco, CA: Berrett-Kohler Publishers, Inc.

de Villiers, M. R., and C. Naidoo. 2011. The consultation—a different approach to the patient: The patient-centered clinical method. In B. Mash, ed., *Handbook of family medicine*, 3rd edition. Cape Town: Oxford University Press.

Frenk, J., L. Chen, Z. A. Bhutta, J. Cohen, N. Crisp, T. Evans, H. Fineberg, P. Garcia, Y. Ke, P. Kelley, B. Kistnasamy, A. Meleis, D. Naylor, A. Pablos-Mendez, S. Reddy, S. Scrimshaw, J. Sepulveda, and H. Zuraykl. 2010. Health professionals for a new century: Transforming education to strengthen health systems in an interdependent world. *Lancet* 376(9756):1923–1958.

Hagopian, A., A. Zuyderduin, N. Kyobutungi, and F. Yumkella. 2009. Job satisfaction and morale in the Ugandan health workforce. *Health Affairs* 28(5):863–875.

Hofstede, G., G. J. Hofstede, and M. Minkov. 2010. *Cultures and organizations: Software of the mind*, 3rd edition. New York: McGraw-Hill.

Interprofessional Education Collaborative Expert Panel. 2011. *Core competencies for interprofessional collaborative practice: Report of an expert panel.* Washington, DC: Interprofessional Education Collaborative.

IOM (Institute of Medicine). 2003. *Health Professions Education: A bridge to quality.* Washington, DC: The National Academies Press.

IOM. 2011. *The future of nursing: Leading change, advancing health.* Washington, DC: The National Academies Press.

Kern, D., P. Thomas, and M. Hughes, eds. 2009. *Curriculum development for medical education: A six-step approach*, 2nd edition. Baltimore, MD: The Johns Hopkins Press.

Kiguli, S., R. Baingana, L. Paina, D. Mafigiri, S. Groves, G. Katende, E. Kiguli-Malwadde, J. Kiguli, M. Galukande, M. Roy, R. Bollinger, and G. Pariyo. 2011. Situational analysis of teaching and learning of medicine and nursing students at Makerere University College of Health Sciences. *BMC International Health and Human Rights* 11(Suppl 1):S3.

Kizza, I., J. Tugumisirize, R. Tweheyo, S. Mbabali, A. Kasangaki, E. Nshimye, J. Sekandi, S. Groves, and C. E. Kennedy. 2011. Makerere University College of Health Sciences' role in addressing challenges in health service provision at Mulago National Referral Hospital. *BMC International Health and Human Rights* 11(Suppl 1):S7.

Pearce, C. L., C. C. Manz, and H. P. Sims. 2009. Where do we go from here? Is shared leadership the key to team success? *Organizational Dynamics* 38(3):234–238.

Rath, T., and B. Conchie. 2008. *Strengths based leadership.* New York: Gallup Press.

Royal College of Physicians. 2005. *Doctors in society: Medical professionalism in a changing world.* London, UK: Working Party of the Royal College of Physicians of London.

UNHCO (Uganda National Health Consumers' Organisation). 2003. *Study on patient feedback mechanisms at health facilities in Uganda.* Kampala, Uganda: UNHCO.

UNHCO. 2010. *Establishing incidence of health provider absenteeism in Bushenyi District.* Kampala, Uganda: UNHCO.

Wilkinson, T. J., W. B. Wade, and L. D. Knock. 2009. A blueprint to assess professionalism: Results of a systematic review. *Academic Medicine* 84:551–558.

D

Faculty Development Programs at Various Universities

Institution	Program	Description
Grand Valley State University, Office of the Vice Provost for Health	E-360 Faculty Development Center	One of the interprofessional resources developed by the Office of the Vice Provost for Health is the faculty, staff, and student interprofessional collaborative practice (IPCP) program. This program is available online in the E-360 Learning Management System (LMS). The faculty development IPCP program includes pre/post tests for each of the following modules: IPE Faculty Development, A Learner's Introduction to IPE & Collaborative Practice, Patient Safety, Team Dynamics, and an IP Preceptor Manual Overview, surveys, and program evaluation materials. These modules increase awareness of IPCP and promote cross-cultural competence development.
		A learning culture is developed through daily huddles and the promotion of sharing disciplinary knowledge, fostering teamwork, and demonstrating appreciation of other team members. Daily Huddle Guidelines to provide structure to the team huddle sessions have been developed. Huddles are used to evaluate and improve team-based patient care while offering an opportunity to build interprofessional communication skills. Useful in guiding patient-practitioner collaboration is an integrative care plan template that has been developed as an additional resource for faculty, staff, and students.
		A resource that is available to faculty and preceptors is the *Interprofessional Preceptor Manual*. The manual is designed to support interprofessional education (IPE) in clinical settings for students, preceptors, and academic faculty. It also provides guidelines for facilitating IPE and interprofessional care learning experiences for students.

Institution	Program	Description
Grand Valley State University, Office of the Vice Provost for Health	Lunch & Learn Series	From October 20, 2012, through April 2013 the Office of the Vice Provost for Health has hosted a monthly Lunch & Learn series for staff and faculty. The goal of the Lunch & Learn series has been to provide interprofessional continuing education for a variety of topics ranging from in-situ simulations to using technology to advance interprofessional practices. The intent of the series was to provide continued opportunities for collaboration and skill development in interprofessional education and practice. For any faculty or staff unable to attend the sessions in person, a video of each session is available on the E-360 LMS (learning hub).
	Annual Interprofessional Education Conference	Each year the West Michigan Interprofessional Education Initiative hosts a regional conference to promote IPCP activities. Speakers include national and international experts, and all faculty, staff, students, and community interprofessional partners are invited to attend. The sixth annual IPE conference, Obtaining the Highest Quality at the Lowest Cost: The Case for Interprofessional Education and Practice, will be held September 19–20, 2013.
Medical University of South Carolina (MUSC)	Creating Collaborative Care	MUSC offers the following: (1) an annual interprofessional institute for faculty and professional staff that focuses on interprofessional collaborative skills and leadership for application in educational, research, and clinical settings; (2) an interprofessional education teaching series for faculty interested in enhancing teaching skills specific to interprofessional education; (3) information to community-based preceptors about our interprofessional education program for students; (4) small grants ($15,000) for pilot projects to advance interprofessional education, research, or clinical care at the institution; and (5) a year-long faculty fellowship (the Maralynne D. Mitcham Fellowship) for focused work in interprofessional collaborative practice and education. Presently we are creating a website for our community-based preceptors with more robust information about interprofessional education, including teaching and collaborative practice tips, and we are conducting faculty development with preceptors through workshops and practice-based interventions.

Institution	Program	Description
University of Toronto	Faculty and professional development programs	The ehpic™ (educating health professionals for interprofessional care) program was created in 2005 to develop educators, clinicians, and leaders in interprofessional education, with the knowledge, skills, and attitudes to teach learners and fellow colleagues the art and science of working collaboratively for patient-centered care. This 5-day accredited program has more than graduates from across North America and several international organizations. The Collaborative Change Leadership (CCL) program was created in 2009 for mid-level executives in health care and health education who lead change throughout organizations and across the continuum of care. This 10-month accredited program enables participants to develop, implement, and evaluate a project or strategy within their organization that creates a broad culture shift and sustainable change in priority areas such as interprofessional care, interprofessional education, patient safety, quality, and patient-centered care.
The Safety-Net Clinics	A series of seminars and workshops	The Safety-Net Clinics respond to the challenge of getting faculty to understand the tasks, responsibilities, and actions of other disciplines. Their year-long programs address this challenge by inviting faculty to learn about what other disciplines are doing. These events are tailored after the Health Resources and Services Administration Patient Safety and Clinical Pharmacy Services Collaborative, which focuses on the integration of pharmacy services into patient care and runs a series of learning sessions and action periods for teams to learn together.

Institution	Program	Description
Thomas Jefferson University JCIPE (Jefferson InterProfessional Education Center)	IPE Faculty Development Workshop	Thomas Jefferson University hosts a free intensive writing workshop for faculty twice per year. According to workshop speaker Elizabeth Speakman, participants spend 2 days developing and working on a manuscript that is ready to be implemented. The university also hosts an IPE immersion program twice per year that is open to academics outside of Jefferson. Participating teams create an idea, which they transform and develop into an IPE project ready for implementation. Jefferson faculty groups are given $1,000 without restrictions to implement their projects and get them fully running. Additionally, JCIPE holds a health mentor facilitator workshop each semester for faculty who will be facilitating an interprofessional student group of students assigned to a community health mentor. This workshop provides faculty with tools to function as an effective small group leader using instructional guides and relevant reading material along with face-to-face and recorded sessions on debriefing. Novice facilitators are paired with seasoned facilitators, and satisfaction as well as student surveys are obtained and shared with facilitators to use for planning future sessions.

Institution	Program	Description
University of Arizona	IPEP (Interprofessional Education and Practice)	Alongside their work building a longitudinal curriculum, the Arizona Area Health Education Center (AzAHEC)–funded IPEP program is building a faculty development program. Faculty and preceptors receive training on how to mentor teams of students from multiple health professions. In spring 2012 IPEP piloted three faculty-preceptor training workshops dealing with teams and teamwork, communication, and teaching interprofessionally. These trainings will be available for organizations that wish to host interprofessional teams of students in the future.
	Arizona Area Health Education Centers Program (AzAHEC)	The AzAHEC has launched an interprofessional academic fellowship program in clinical outcomes and comparative effectiveness research (the COCER program). The COCER Fellowship Program is a 2-year career development program funding four doctorally prepared fellows per year from four health care disciplines: family and community medicine (M.D.), nursing (D.N.P.), pharmacy (Pharm.D.), and public health (Ph.D. or Dr.P.H.). About 80 percent of the fellows' time is spent in research training, collaborative research projects at the T3 and T4 translational levels, and a mentored research project. The AzAHEC supports the IPEP, as the remaining 20 percent of fellows' time is devoted to interprofessional primary care practice in environments that serve underserved, predominantly rural populations in the Tucson area.
	Arizona Center on Aging	The Arizona Center on Aging presents an interprofessional 160-hour Faculty Scholars in Aging Program for professionals in public health, nursing, medicine, nurse practitioners, physician assistants, social work, pharmacy, and psychology faculty in collaboration with the Arizona Geriatric Education Center.

Institution	Program	Description
University of British Columbia, Canada (UBC)	IPE collaborative learning series	At the UBC there is an interprofessional collaborative learning series based on the Institute for Healthcare Improvement (IHI) principles. This involves going out to the health authorities to actually do development with both preceptors and practitioners. In addition, there is a focus on faculty development for preceptors and creating interprofessional learning experiences for the students that are out in practice as the students at UBC spend almost 50 percent of their time or more in the practice environment.
University of California, San Francisco (UCSF)	Courses in faculty development for IPE	UCSF offers two courses for faculty development in IPE: (1) The Challenge of Providing Quality Care for Older Adults: Preparing the Health Professions for the Aging Century, and (2) New Interprofessional Education and Practice Workshop Series.
University of Missouri	Achieving Competence Today (ACT) initiative	As part of the ACT initiative, faculty and health workers undergo interprofessional training with the health professions students, covering issues such as quality improvement skills, interprofessional education, and an error disclosure program that was recently adapted from the University of Washington.
University of New England		Faculty development is part of strategic plan at the University of New England. It includes training each year, participating in TeamSTEPPS training, working to become a TeamSTEPPS site, bringing in outside experts, and establishing mentors for faculty.

Institution	Program	Description
University of Virginia (UVA)	Faculty development and clinician continuing IPE programs	Many UVA faculty members and clinicians are directly involved in using the collaborative care best practices model approach, which brings them together for continuing interprofessional education and supports them in developing, implementing, and assessing their own new IPE experiences for students, residents, and clinicians. Formal continuing IPE programs are offered at UVA, and many faculty members have been sponsored to attend external programs such as the Macy Foundation Faculty Development in Team-Based Care and Collaborating Across Borders. IPE consultants provide small-group faculty development seminars as well as health system–wide presentations. Other faculty and clinician development programs for IPE include the School of Medicine speakers series, appreciative practices workshops, quality and safety workshops, error disclosure workshops, Schwarz rounds, and the Virginia Geriatric Education Consortium series. A new website will offer many resources for self-directed IPE faculty and clinician development.
Department of Veterans Affairs (VA)	VA centers of excellence in primary care education	One example of the VA's work includes bringing in the University of Toronto Center for IPE for faculty development exercises. Another VA site has developed a huddle coaching program for its faculty and students. All sites are using the team development measure to look at interprofessional collaboration.

Institution	Program	Description
Western University of Health Sciences (WesternU)	Small-group IPE faculty training	Because of the curricular design of its IPE program, there are 130 facilitated small groups that meet for 10 2-hour sessions throughout the academic year. WesternU currently operates two campuses. The main campus is located in Pomona, California, and a second campus with only an osteopathic medical college is located in Lebanon, Oregon. The IPE curriculum is delivered in an inter-institutional model with students and faculty also participating from Oregon State University and Linn-Benton Community College near the campus in Oregon. A modified problem-based learning method of course delivery is used, and it requires faculty who are trained and comfortable conducting these small group sessions. All faculty who facilitate in the IPE program receive annual facilitator development training. Approximately 250 faculty attend training sessions each academic year. Content includes the history and basis of IPE and collaborative care. It also includes small group teaching and learning, and facilitating student-centered learning activities. Additionally, faculty may attend optional monthly facilitator continuing education sessions throughout the year. Issues related to the implementation of the IPE program are discussed, and specific facilitation skills are emphasized.
	Professional scope of practice training	There are 13 health professions represented and more than 200 faculty who participate in the delivery of the IPE curriculum. To maximize faculty effectiveness, a scope of practice faculty learning experience has been developed and is offered to all faculty members at several times throughout the year. These sessions are conducted as small workshops where participants are actively engaged in completing a template used to describe similarities and differences among scopes of practice of all 13 professions. While it does not include all practice act content, participants do benefit by describing what they know about various professions while learning many things that they did not know. Using this approach, the training is applicable to seasoned clinicians as well as to basic scientists without a clinical background.

Institution	Program	Description
University of Washington	Web-based modules for faculty instructors	With funding from the Macy Foundation and the Health Resources and Services Administration, the University of Washington provides IPE Faculty Development programs that involve eight academic centers. The university's Center for Health Science Interprofessional Education, Research, and Practice has developed a website to serve as a resource for faculty that centralizes the university's IPE faculty development programs and opportunities, including Web-based modules on topics such as teaching with simulation, computing and technology fundamentals, and distance learning. The website is available at http://collaborate.uw.edu/faculty-development/faculty-development.html.

E

Disruptive Innovations

Area of IPE	Program/Idea	Description
Curricular innovations Concentrates on *what* is being taught to health professions learners to meet evolving domestic and international needs	Faculty sharing	Lorna Lynn from the American Board of Internal Medicine presented for her "Better Care" small group. She echoed a common theme of needing greater faculty development but then went on to introduce a new concept. The idea is "faculty sharing." In this scheme any school or university could use skills and knowledge of any faculty member in any school in order to promote educational understanding of interprofessional education (IPE).

Area of IPE	Program/Idea	Description
	Global collaborative leadership model	The idea is to co-create, develop, and implement a global collaborative leadership model. This model builds on relationships among the South Africa Collaborative, the collaborative in Uganda, and the Indian Collaborative and aims to enhance the cultural applicability of a leadership curriculum. The hope is to apply the lessons learned from each of the country collaboratives about the various ways of addressing and teaching leadership to students and health professionals (see Appendix C for details on the country collaboratives).
Pedagogic innovations Looks at *how* the information can be better taught to students and *where* education can take place	Pass/fail curriculums	In his remarks about trust, Sandeep Kishore, who represented health professional students, observed that a culture of trust on university campuses has given way to stereotypes of competitive students sabotaging the work of fellow learners. He thinks the grading system is one of the triggers preventing collaboration that could be addressed through pass/fail curriculums at the university level.

Area of IPE	Program/Idea	Description
	Jeffersonian dinners	Tina Brashers and other IPE educators from the University of Virginia (UVA) created a social space through what is known at UVA as a Jeffersonian dinner. At this honorific event, key students are invited to sit down with a group of roughly 10 educators to talk through ideas on how the professions could work more effectively together.
	Hub-and-spoke model	Mark Earnest at the University of Colorado recognized early on the daunting task of trying to train every clinical preceptor to be an IPE preceptor. As a result, he and his colleagues adopted a "hub-and-spoke" model in which a single preceptor monitors multiple teams working in different settings. When the teams are in their settings, they typically work with their profession-specific preceptors. Following the experience, teams reconvene with the IPE preceptor, who reviews the process with the students. In this model, students learn by experiencing negative as well as positive examples. One of the goals at the University of Colorado is to help learners stay focused on positive examples of collaboration and to become agents of change when the situation dictates a need for greater collaboration. Dawn Forman at Curtin University in Australia also uses the hub-and-spoke model.

Area of IPE	Program/Idea	Description
Cultural elements Addresses *who* is being taught by whom as a means of enhancing the effectiveness of the design, development, and implementation of interprofessional health professional education	Service learning model	In her summary remarks, Forum member Madeline Schmitt noted that the service learning model gets students into the community and gets them there early. But she also pointed out that speakers often found that service learning is disconnected from the clinical experiences that come afterward. In Uganda, where service learning and social accountability are used as an organizing framework for the curriculum, when students go into their clinical experiences, the IPE drops off. Linking IPE and service throughout the continuum of health professional education is a tool for achieving a person-centered perspective. Service learning is a concept that Marietjie de Villiers from South Africa compared to the "helicopter model." As she says, "We shouldn't be coming in and providing care. We should be integrating and understanding and learning from the patients and from the people within the community."

Area of IPE	Program/Idea	Description
	Patients as educators	According to Sally Okun from PatientsLikeMe, trust begins with acknowledging the importance of patient engagement. By partnering with patients, providers and learners gain a better understanding of the needs and concerns of the populations and individuals they are serving. Through better alignment, providers, learners, and patients build trust that can lead to shared values, such as improved use of technology and patient empowerment through data. These data can be generated by patients themselves and shared with students and providers once trust is established.

Area of IPE	Program/Idea	Description
Human resources for health Focuses on *how* capacity can be innovatively expanded to better ensure an adequate supply and mix of educated health workers based on local needs	Community colleges	Forum member Warren Newton commented on the cost of U.S. education and perhaps also education in the United Kingdom. This is an unprecedented period of time and change when higher education is being fiscally driven and is experiencing challenges similar to those in medicine with regard to cost, quality, and patient (or student) experience, he said. Community colleges may be one solution to the fiscal obstacles to education. In the United States, 40 percent of adults in higher education are in community colleges. It's where the new professions that will be needed to transform education will come from in addition to the traditional educational systems. Today's professional and educational leaders need to understand this broader context when discussing practice redesign.
Metrics Addresses *how* one measures whether learner assessments and the evaluation of educational impact and care delivery systems influence individual and population health.	MedEdPORTAL	Forum member Carol Aschenbrener who is with the Association of American Medical Colleges received funding from the Macy Foundation to develop an IPE portal on the MedEdPORTAL platform. On this website there is a section for non-peer-reviewed publications called iCollaborative, where anyone can submit ideas and share thoughts on activities under way at their institutions.

Area of IPE	Program/Idea	Description
	Value-added learners	In an effort to integrate learners into Colorado Children's Hospital, students of Mark Earnest, the director of interprofessional education at the University of Colorado, gathered requested data for the hospital. This is a cost savings for the hospital and an educational bonus for students, who are no longer seen as a burden to the system.
	Student educators	Mark Earnest also organizes students to assess how well the hospital teams function. After receiving proper training, the students then observe those clinical teams that volunteered for the activity. Following the observation, feedback is provided to the teams on how they might improve their teamwork.